Managing Emergency Medical Services:
Principles and Practices

William L. Newkirk, M.D.
Richard P. Linden, M.B.A.

Reston Publishing Company, Inc.
A Prentice-Hall Company
Reston, Virginia

Library of Congress Cataloging in Publication Data

Newkirk, William L.
  Managing emergency medical services:
  principles and practices

  Includes bibliographical references.
    1. Hospitals—Emergency service—Administration.
I. Linden, Richard P. II. Title. [DNLM: 1. Emergency
medical services—Organization and administration.
WX 215 N548m]
RA975.5.E5N49 1984   362.1′8′068   83–24582
ISBN 0–8359–4198–1

© 1984 by Reston Publishing Company, Inc.
A Prentice-Hall Company
Reston, Virginia 22090

10   9   8   7   6   5   4   3   2   1

Printed in the United States of America

This book is dedicated to our parents.

Contents

Preface

EMS managers at all levels within the EMS system helped us write this book. They came from urban centers and country towns, advanced and basic ambulance services, teaching centers and community hospitals. They worked as EMTs, physicians, nurses, and administrators. We've listed some of their names in our acknowledgments. However, most of the managers who spoke with us did so confidentially, and we are deeply indebted to them–without them, this book would not exist.

When we talked with these successful EMS managers, we could see in their eyes the toll that years of work in EMS had taken. They had become effective EMS managers, often learning their management lessons the hard way. It is a tribute to their endurance and commitment that they survived frequent failure to make EMS what it is today.

It was their hope, and ours, that we could begin learning from each other's triumphs and defeats; that new EMS managers would be better prepared as managers than many of us were; and that by working together, we could continue the development of EMS.

W. L. N.
R. P. L.

Acknowledgments

We would specifically like to thank the following people for their help with this book: Nancy Aubin, Chester Baker, Dr. Pamela Bensen, Audrey Blaisdell, T. J. Brown, Dr. Marshall Chamberlain, Bruce Cummings, Thea Fickett, Herb Flint, Dr. Bruce Hutson, Frank Keegan, Dr. Benjamin Linden, Dr. Sidney Miller, Dr. Maurice Newkirk, Ruth Newkirk, D. Anne Paquet, Marcia Paton, Dr. Paul Reinstein, Dr. Larry Ricci, Dr. Mark Silver, Bernard Spooner, Doris Sylvester, Dr. William Taggart, Patty Van Horne, and Jimmie Woodlee.

We would like to thank Mabel Larsen for her help with Chapters 3 and 9, Dana Kempton for Chapter 4, and Michael Keller and Gary Snowden for Chapter 10.

We would like to thank Pat Cote and Barbara Woodlee for their help in our understanding EMS education.

We would like to thank the members of the Kennebec Valley Regional EMS Council, the Redington-Fairview EMS committee, and the Menorah Medical Center for their assistance. We would like to thank the students in our management courses and our fellow EMS personnel who gave us insight into "real world" EMS management problems.

We wish to thank Joan Hart, managing editor of *Emergency Medical Services*, for her encouragement and willingness to publish articles on EMS management.

We wish to thank Jane Washburn and Donna Pomelow for their assistance in preparing this manuscript.

Our editor at Reston Publishing, Barbara Lovenvirth, played a major role in creating this book.

We wish to thank Benjamin MacArthur for insight and guidance in management areas.

We wish to thank Thomas Harmelink for his thorough reviewing of the manuscript, and for his very helpful suggestions.

We wish to thank the dedicated members of the Redington-Fairview General Hospital Emergency Medical System, who filled out endless forms, answered a barrage of questions, and contributed greatly to the conclusions in this book. Without their high-spirited cooperation, we could not have investigated many of the questions we did.

Above all, we would like to thank our beautiful wives, whose criticism made this book better and whose support made this book possible.

Introduction

Do you manage all or part of an emergency medical system (EMS)? If so, this book is for you. It is for emergency medical technicians (EMTs) who manage ambulance services, physicians who direct emergency departments, nurses who supervise critical care areas, and administrators who manage EMS systems. If you manage in emergency medicine, you already know the high stress and risks involved. If you plan to manage, you'd better know them. If you want to manage effectively, there's much that you need to know. That's where this book comes in.

Why do some EMS managers succeed while others fail? There are several pitfalls, and this book will alert you to them. The fundamental reason for failure is that most nurses, doctors, and EMTs who manage in emergency medicine were never trained as managers. Here is an example of what often happens: An EMT develops increasingly effective patient care skills. In time, extrication, IVs, and cardiac dysrhythmias become a snap. Then that EMT is promoted to EMS supervisor. Suddenly the EMT is in strange territory. Instead of providing direct patient care, he is negotiating, supervising, planning, and educating. Without training in these areas the EMT makes mistakes, creates problems, becomes frustrated, and ultimately fails. It's all so unnecessary. Starting IVs had to be learned; so does management.

Effective management techniques exist. Most of the techniques have been developed in nonmedical fields—business, government, and the military. This book will show you how these techniques apply to emergency medical services and how they can be made to work for you. In addition, successful EMS managers have developed management techniques that address specific problems in EMS. We'll discuss those techniques, too, and how you can use them.

In this book we've divided EMS management into five elements: planning, organizing, directing, controlling, and surviving. In Section I, "Planning," you'll learn to develop goals, both personal and organizational. You'll learn time management techniques for protecting your valuable time, directing you toward what you really want out of life, and teaching you how to achieve the best organizational results with reasonable effort. Planning is perhaps the most critical phase in management; after all, if you don't know where you're heading, you'll never arrive there.

In Section II, "Organizing," you'll learn how to allocate your resources—both human and financial—to achieve your established goals. This step is important if you are to use your resources effectively (so as to achieve desired results) and efficiently (so that you don't needlessly waste your resources in the process).

In Section III, "Directing," you'll develop skills that will enable you to achieve your goals using your organized resources. You'll learn listening skills that will save you from failing to hear small problems before they mushroom into crises, and assertiveness skills that will enable you to deal with difficult situations without "losing your cool." You'll become a better negotiator and delegator and develop skills that will help you manage change.

In Section IV, "Controlling," you'll compare the actual results that you achieve with the expectations that you developed during the planning and organizing phases. These comparisons will enable you to determine if your service is operating as you intended. If you uncover deviations from what you expected, you can then take corrective action.

As a manager, you must survive. If you have been managing emergency medical services for very long, you have seen other managers cracking under the strain and burning out. You must avoid a similar fate. This book can help you. In Section V, "Surviving," you'll learn about stress: what it is, how it affects you, and how you can control it. What you are going to learn, to your delight, is that techniques that help to protect you as a manager also produce excellent organizational results. You'll find yourself better prepared to face challenges and produce positive results.

No one said that this would be easy. But, if you wanted the easy way out, you wouldn't have chosen a career in EMS. We've chosen to dedicate our lives to a stressful, emotionally charged field. EMS management can be extremely difficult. But, like starting IVs, it can be learned. Once you've mastered the skills, your life as a manager will be easier, more productive, and more rewarding. So let's get started.

PLANNING

I

To be an effective EMS manager, the first area that you must master is planning. You must be able to plan successfully your time, life, and work. This section contains two chapters. Chapter 1, "Planning Your Life and Your Work," will introduce you to techniques for goal setting and time management. Chapter 2, "Planning for Your EMS Organization," will demonstrate how you can apply organizational planning techniques to EMS.

Planning your life and your work

I don't manage my time as well as I should. I admire the manager who has his goals spelled out clearly and sticks to them so that he can look back in a month or six weeks and check off what he has accomplished. I tend to respond to the squeaky wheel. I let other people manage my time. As a result, I have trouble carrying tasks through to completion. I end up with a desk full of half-completed projects.
—STATE EMS OFFICIAL

Time management has never been a hot subject in EMS management.[1] If you've managed in EMS any length of time, you've probably spent many more hours discussing disasters or defibril-
lators than you have discussing time management. Yet we are
starting this book with time management. If you burn out, you're
not going to be much help to anyone. As a manager, you must
realize that your time is one of your service's most important resources. Some managers will work hard to save a few dollars on
the purchase of new equipment, thinking that they are conserv-
ing their service's financial resources, then turn around and
squander hours of their time sitting in meaningless, nonproduc-
tive meetings. Your time is often more valuable than money.
Don't waste it.

Are you an effective time-manager? To find out, ask yourself
these questions. In the last year, have you

- Said, "If you want something done right, do it yourself?"
- Had to miss an important event in your personal life because you had work commitments?
- Felt tense or anxious because you didn't have time for all
  that was expected of you?
- Promised yourself that next month or next year you
  would begin that project that was really important to
  you?
- Thought you worked too hard and accomplished too little?

If you answered yes to any of these questions, chances are that
you have time management problems. Don't worry—you're not
alone.

Useful time is in short supply for most EMS managers. The
development of EMS has created a broad range of grants, programs, committees, and commitments that demand your time. In
addition, many managers provide direct patient care, which uses
up more time. Unfortunately this situation is likely to worsen.
With each month bringing new demands, you must learn to manage time effectively or burn out racing to meet all the new
demands. Effective time management thus becomes a matter of
survival.

EMS managers often resist time management because they
equate it with time-motion studies designed to make a person a

more productive assembly-line worker or a swifter paper pusher. Any effort that enables you to do meaningless tasks more efficiently so that you can do more meaningless tasks is absurd. That's not time management.

Time management is actually a misnomer. Time is never managed; it is always moving forward. You couldn't stop it if you wanted. What you control is how you behave relative to time. Thus time management is really self-management. In order to manage EMS effectively, you must first learn to manage yourself. Effective time management can begin only when you understand that to be a successful manager, you must balance your personal, work, and organizational goals. This requires that you learn to allocate time more effectively. By selecting tasks designed to produce the greatest impact you can actually improve your effectiveness as a manager while reducing your time commitments. In this way, time management can produce not only a better-managed EMS system but also a happier, more rested, burnout-proof manager.

Learning the importance of planning

Let's go meet someone. If you've been in EMS management very long, you've probably seen this person once or twice. When you walk into his office, the first thing you notice is how serious he is. "Listen," he says looking up from his desk, "I've got two meetings this evening and I've got a lot to do. Someone has to care about this place." He's convinced how important he is to his organization. Notice how cluttered his desk is. "I'd like to straighten it up," he says, restacking some papers for the fifth time, "but I really don't have the time, and anyway, I've got several projects that I've got to watch very carefully." You can't help noticing how tired he looks. "May I be frank with you," he says, glancing around to see if anyone else is listening. "If I didn't work my tail off, this place would go downhill in a hurry. You can count on that!"

You look around and see his briefcase, which is crammed so full of papers that it can't be closed. He sees you looking at it. "You see," he says, "that's just some of the work that I need to do. I don't want it fouled up, so I'm going to do it at home." You realize that with all this important work his home life must be deteriorating. "I haven't noticed any problems," he says. You wonder whether he has time to notice. He looks as if he needs a vacation. His family would love it. "A vacation," he laughs. "Do you know what would happen if I left this place? The people here wouldn't last a week." He glances at his watch. "I'm sorry, but I really have to get back to work." Let's leave.

That is the ineffective workaholic.[2] Many EMS managers turn into ineffective workaholics. Constantly in motion, forever on edge, and hopelessly ineffective, the workaholic is a self-appointed martyr. When approached with ideas about the importance of planning and time management, the workaholic looks up from the desk, says that the ideas sound fine, but has no time for them.

Planning is essential if you are to avoid the trap of becoming an ineffective workaholic, with a calendar full of meaningless, low-priority activities that cripple effectiveness. If you don't plan your organization's future, you'll float like a rudderless ship moving in whatever direction the wind is blowing. If you don't plan your work, you'll run into countless, frustrating delays that could have been avoided if you had only taken the time to think. But above all, if you don't plan your life, you'll waste it.

Planning is the key. As an EMS manager, if you don't plan, be prepared to fail. Planning is the essence of management. You plot the course and determine what you need to do to arrive there. To one unaccustomed to time management, the thought of setting aside a day to plan a project may seem like a waste of time. Experience shows, however, that time spent in planning is recouped manyfold.

Even though planning will save time and help ensure that goals are achieved, most EMS managers don't plan effectively. Nowhere is that more apparent than in the most important area of planning—the manager's personal life.

Planning your life

Seven years of conducting seminars on setting life goals for EMS personnel reveals a startling lack of planning by EMS managers. Before the seminars fewer than 10 percent of the managers had given any concrete thought to what their life goals were and how they should attempt to reach them. Because this step is essential for effective time management, the magnitude of the problem represented by this fact is staggering: 90 percent of EMS managers don't know where they are going in their personal lives.

The lack of personal life goals is a major pitfall in EMS management. Now is the time for you to avoid that pitfall by setting your life goals. Don't put it off, or you'll just invite failure.

The seminars on setting life goals follow an exercise developed by Alan Lakein, a noted expert on time management.[3] The exercise enables participants to establish realistic life goals. Take out a piece of paper and pencil and complete the exercise that follows.

STEP 1. Looking at your personal, social, family, professional, financial, community, and spiritual goals, write down your life goals in each area. Make the list as all-inclusive as possible. Feel free to write down any goal even if it seems unattainable or ridiculous. What do you really want out of life? Do you want to write a Top 10 song, be president of the Elks Club, be the local tennis champion, have six children? Remember that you're just writing these things down on paper, not etching them into marble. So be loose and write fast.

STEP 2. Repeat the same exercise, but now make the time frame three years. These goals will probably be a little more specific.

STEP 3. Now we get a little morbid. If you knew that you were going to be struck dead by lightning in six months, how would you live until then? (Assume that someone will attend to all the details of your death and funeral.)

STEP 4. Think about this: If you knew that you were going to die, you would probably do only those things that really matter to you in life. You wouldn't waste your time. If your response to step 3 was much different from your responses to steps 1 and 2, then you have a conflict. If you would do something completely different with your life if you knew that you were going to die soon, then perhaps your life goals do not reflect what you really want. Often at this point people say: "Well, if I knew I were going to die, I'd do things that really matter to me, but I can't do that all the time. After all, I have responsibilities." Sure, we all have responsibilities. But nothing says that our jobs and responsibilities can't be consistent with what we really want in life. After all, if you are not going to pursue the things that you really want in life, during your life, when are you going to pursue them?

STEP 5. Revise your answers until you are satisfied that they reflect as much as possible what you really want from life. Then prioritize each list. On another sheet of paper write: "My three most important life goals are...." List the top three responses. Do this for three-year and six-month goals also.

STEP 6. Recognize two things. First, these goals are not static; they must be revised periodically. Second, with proper time management there is no reason why you can't start working on your most preferred activity today.

What have seven years of life-goals–setting seminars taught us about EMS managers?

First, EMS managers rarely mention the organization for which they work within their long-term goals. Managers see their employers and jobs as means to achieve personal goals and not as ends in themselves.

Second, in the first draft, the managers' life and three-year goals are usually substantially different from the managers' goals if death were imminent. This means that there is likely to be a great deal of difference between what the EMS managers initially think they want out of life and what they find out they really want.

Third, and most important, long-term goals usually reflect such things as health, family, free time, and happiness. These findings are often a direct contradiction of the way the EMS manager is living—working long hours under high stress with little time or energy for recreation or family. When one considers this great discrepancy between personal needs and professional behavior, is it a surprise that so many EMS managers burn out?

What did you learn from determining your life goals? Are you like most managers, learning that long hours spent in a succession of insignificant meetings is not the way you want to live your life? Realize that since you now understand your life goals, you are better prepared than 90 percent of EMS managers. You have formed the basis for rational time management. If you decided to put off doing this exercise until you had more time or decided that you were different from all other managers and didn't really need to define your life goals, put this book down and stop reading. You *can't* manage effectively unless you know where you're going.

Proper time management allows you to pursue personal life goals. Once you have recognized the importance of planning, established your life goals, and understood the great difference that often exists between life goals and professional behavior, you can begin to reevaluate your work. By applying time-management principles to your job, you can become a more effective manager while still meeting personal needs.

When looking at your job, you must be a realist. You will inevitably have conflicts between your work and your personal life. By applying time management principles, you can reduce that conflict, but you can't eliminate it. In addition, you are likely to have conflicts between your work goals and the goals of your organization. For example, you might think that the wisest use of your time is to attend a disaster planning meeting, while your boss thinks that you should stay at home and work a shift on the ambulance.

As you become a more effective manager, these conflicts are likely to increase. For example, as your service becomes more successful, you will be asked to speak to more outside groups. This is likely to create conflicts with your family life. Which is more important: speaking to a regional EMS meeting or going to a birthday party with your daughter? Often you will be unable to satisfy everyone.

Planning your work

Establishing work goals

When you apply time management concepts to your work, you need to establish goals that are consistent with your organization's goals. This makes sense because it's important that your work fits into your organization's overall plan. For completing your work goals, you should set a time frame that is long enough so that you can complete the goals but short enough that you receive frequent feedback on your progress. If you don't have any experience in establishing work goals, you might try one year as an initial time frame.

You need to write down and prioritize your work goals. Writing down goals is important because it forces you to define what you are trying to do. Some goals are unclear: You may think

all around them but never put your finger on them unless forced
to by writing them down. Because you will rarely complete unde-
fined goals, you must define your goals clearly before proceeding
further.

To illustrate the techniques of setting work goals, imagine
that you are the director of an ambulance service. Like many ambulance service directors you have money problems, political
problems, personnel problems, and equipment problems. You're
beginning to wonder why you entered EMS in the first place.
Looking ahead to the next year, you list seven goals:

- Improve staffing on second ambulance.
- Increase number of runs.
- Expand area covered by the service.
- Purchase a new ambulance.
- Improve relations with the local hospital emergency de-
  partment.
- Develop a regional disaster plan.
- Solve problems with radio communications south of
  town.

All these goals are important to you, but you probably won't have
time to accomplish them all in the next year. As a result, once you
have developed your goals, you must prioritize them. Unless you
prioritize your goals, they will become one large soup from
which you randomly serve yourself. The likelihood of spending
your time on your most important goals will be only as high as
the likelihood of spending your time on your least important
goals. Your time is too valuable to rely on such a random process.

One way to prioritize your goals is to label your most important goals A, less important goals B, and least important goals C.
In fact, prioritizing is so important that you should further prioritize your A goals into A1, A2, A3, etc. This process leaves no
doubt about where you should concentrate your time.

Returning to our example, as the director of an ambulance
service, you need to prioritize your work goals:

- Improve staffing on second ambulance. (A2. Current
  staffing should hold out for a few months, but when vacations start, there will be real problems.)
- Increase number of runs. (C. Would be desirable, particularly if staffing problems are solved.)

11

- Expand area covered by the service. (A3. Certainly would improve patient care in surrounding regions, but there are political obstacles to doing it.)
- Purchase a new ambulance. (C. It's needed, but there's no money right now.)
- Improve relations with the local hospital emergency department. (A1. Relations have been going downhill for some time. Lately the doctors have been kicking paramedics out of the department.)
- Develop a regional disaster plan. (C. The region needs one, but people aren't working together well enough yet to hope for success.)
- Solve problems with radio communications south of town. (B. The problems have been around for a while, but it looks as if you could solve them.)

Specifying activities

Once you have identified and prioritized your goals, examine each goal in greater depth. Goals are usually too large to complete in one step. For this reason you must follow goal setting with shorter-term planning, where you specify doable activities. This process resembles the goal-setting process and should be closely coordinated with it. Here's how it works:

1. For each goal that you have identified, list all possible activities that can assist in achieving that goal.
2. Prioritize the activities so you can logically choose the most effective activities to do now.
3. Eliminate those activities from your list that will have the least effect on completing the goal.

These three steps result in a realistic list of high-output activities that will direct you toward completing your goals.

Some things are more easily said than done. For example, how do you decide which tasks are most effective in helping you achieve your work goals and which tasks should be avoided? This decision is important if you are to use your time effectively. The Pareto principle helps you make that decision.

Applying the Pareto principle

The Pareto principle, named after the nineteenth century Italian economist and sociologist Vilfredo Pareto, states that in any group of items only a few are significant.[4] Another common name for this is the 80/20 rule, which states that in any given activity 80 percent of the results come from 20 percent of the work. Applying the Pareto principle to time management would indicate that you can achieve substantial results from only a small amount of activity. So to be an effective time manager, you need to identify the key tasks that will produce a disproportionate share of the results and concentrate efforts on completing them.

One of the most important tasks of this kind is the leveraged task, where the completion of one key activity facilitates the completion of numerous other activities. A classic example of a leveraged task is delegation: By spending a few hours training another person to handle certain managerial responsibilities, you can produce hundreds of additional hours of managerial performance. To be an effective time manager, you must use delegation extensively. The statement "if you want something done right, do it yourself" is generally made by a poor time manager. We will discuss delegation in more depth in Chapter 7.

Deciding what not to do

Nobody can do everything. Effective time management requires both the ability to undertake those tasks that are likely to produce significant results and the ability to refuse those tasks that are not time-effective. There are two rules for deciding what not to do:

1. Avoid any task that is likely to produce an insignificant outcome.

There are numerous examples of this in EMS. For example, most EMS organizations form standing committees. Some of these committees meet regularly, discuss mundane matters, and decide little of importance. If committees like these are a drain on your time, avoid them.

"Wait a minute," you say. "That's a pretty strong statement. Aren't you taking a simplistic view of meetings? Meetings often serve as communication channels. As such, they are often valuable resources even though the specific issues discussed may be insignificant." You have a good point. Meetings are often useful for reasons other than their specific purpose. If you can find a useful and important reason for attending a meeting, go to the meeting. The purpose of this rule is to remind you that you shouldn't attend meetings, or do anything else, that is likely to have an insignificant impact. Don't do things out of habit or just because people expect you to do them.

2. Avoid any task that will produce a positive outcome whether you are involved or not.

In these cases you must resist the urge to overmanage. If a personnel problem, given time, is likely to resolve itself, or a committee is certain to recommend a positive course of action, you should sit on the sidelines and let things happen. Good outcomes can occur without your direct involvement.

"Hold on!" you say. "That sounds like a good way to get into trouble. I'm supposed to start ignoring personnel problems and poof, like magic, they'll go away. That's crazy. The only time I'd be comfortable doing that is when I knew what the problem was, how my service was likely to react, and what risks I would be taking in not acting." Again, you're right. This rule does not give you permission to ignore problems. What it does is give you permission to allow problems to work themselves out if you understand the problem and have good reason to believe that a wait-and-watch approach will work.

Let's return to your job as the director of an ambulance service. You need to determine the work activities for your A1 (improve relations with the local hospital emergency department). Possible activities follow:

- Strangle the emergency department physician director.
- Meet with the emergency department nurses.
- Write policies for paramedic behavior in the emergency department.
- Learn how other ambulance services handle relations with the emergency department.
- Schedule a meeting with the emergency department physician director and nursing supervisor.

14

- Meet with the hospital administrator to discuss the problem.

Once you list the activities, you should prioritize them:

- Strangle the emergency department physician director. (C. Impractical.)
- Meet with the emergency department nurses. (B. Making allies of the nurses is important.)
- Write policies for paramedic behavior in the emergency department. (C. Waste of time.)
- Learn how other ambulance services handle relations with the emergency department. (A1. A key first step.)
- Schedule a meeting with the emergency department physician director and nursing supervisor. (A2. Try to learn a little more about the problem.)
- Meet with the hospital administrator to discuss the problem. (B. Might later become an A1.)

So these are the activities that you would pursue at this time:

1. Learn how other ambulance services handle relations with the emergency department.
2. Schedule a meeting with the emergency department physician director and nursing supervisor.
3. Meet with the hospital administrator to discuss the problem.

You should update your activity list periodically. How often you do it is up to you. A monthly review of potential activities for each goal can serve as an excellent vehicle for plotting your work. You can schedule meetings, dispose of little errands, or block out large periods of time to work on your A1. Your planning session will provide you with greater control over your time, but remember to be flexible enough so you can accommodate the unexpected.

In constructing a work schedule you may need to block out large chunks of time for A activities that are not quickly accomplished. Without scheduling a large block of time you may find yourself starting the activity half a dozen times only to run out of time. Schedule the large time block in advance. When that time arrives, treat it with respect. Concentrate your efforts on completing your A activity.

Scheduling your work also enables you to take advantage of your body rhythm. If you think more clearly in the morning than in the afternoon, schedule your large blocks of A1 time during the mornings, when you concentrate best, and pick off those little, necessary-but-annoying details during the afternoons. As long as your taking the time to schedule yourself, you might as well do it as logically and effectively as possible.

Planning your daily work

After you have established your goals and completed your monthly activity sheet to correspond to the goals, you must decide what you are going to do on a daily basis. The following story illustrates the importance of daily planning.[5]

When he was president of Bethlehem Steel, Charles Schwab presented Ivy Lee, a consultant, with an unusual challenge: "Show me a way to get more done with my time," he said, "and I'll pay you any fee within reason."

Handing Schwab a piece of paper, Lee said: "Write down the most important tasks you have to do tomorrow and number them in order of importance. When you arrive in the morning, begin at once on number 1 and stay on it until it's completed. Recheck your priorities; then start on number 2. If a task takes all day, never mind. Stick with it as long as it's the most important one. If you don't finish them all, you probably couldn't have done so with any other method; and without any system, you'd probably not even decide which one of them was most important. Make this a habit every working day. When it works for you, give it to your men. Try it as long as you like. Then send me a check for what you think it's worth."

Some weeks later Schwab sent Lee a check for $25,000 with a note saying that the lesson was the most important he ever learned. In five years the plan was responsible for making Bethlehem Steel the largest independent steel producer in the world. The idea made Schwab $100 million.

The plan that Lee described to Schwab can rarely be applied without changes in EMS. Often there are low-priority tasks that you cannot avoid doing. That's reality. But in general, whether you are making steel or managing EMS, you need to follow this lesson every day:

***Work on the highest priority task possible for as long as
possible every day.***

To ensure that you follow the lesson, you will need to construct a
to-do list on a daily basis. This is best done either at the beginning
of the day or at the end of the preceding day. Whatever time you
choose, be consistent.

The to-do list need not include routine items like opening the
mail. Rather it should include A activities and anything else that
has a high priority today. Some items may be on today's calendar
from prior scheduling. Other items you may have thought of only
today. The important thing is to make the to-do list every day,
keep it visible, and use it as a guide to action as you go through
the day.

It may become apparent as you compose the list that there is
too much to be accomplished in one day. What should be done in
these instances? The answer is obvious. You do what Lee told
Schwab: prioritize your tasks and start on the top priority. One
way to do this is by using the A-B-C method described earlier.
When the work day begins, start with your A1 task. Banish all C
activities during this period. If B or even other A activities rise up
unexpectedly in the form of a potentially long phone call or a visitor and threaten your ability to continue working on your A1, try
to reschedule the phone call or the visitor into a future period. If
you are lucky, the problem may have solved itself by then. Even if
it hasn't, you can probably complete a series of such activities
during that future period.

Let's return to our example. As director of the ambulance
service, the activities that you are pursuing for your A1 goal (improving relations with the emergency department) are as follows:

1.   Learn how other ambulance services handle relations
     with the emergency department.
2.   Schedule a meeting with the emergency department phy-
     sician director and nursing supervisor.
3.   Meet with the hospital administrator to discuss the
     problem.

What can you do today to complete those activities? You could do
these:

  •   Call other ambulance services in the area to gain infor-
      mation.

17

- Write to ambulance services in other areas to determine how they handle problems.
- Call the emergency department physician director and the nursing supervisor to set up an appointment.
- Call the hospital administrator for an appointment.

Now you should prioritize those tasks:

- Call other ambulance services in the area to gain information. (A1. Good idea.)
- Write to ambulance services in other areas to determine how they handle problems. (B. Writing takes time. Hold off for a bit.)
- Call the emergency department physician director and the nursing supervisor to set up an appointment. (A2. Learn about the problems.)
- Call the hospital administrator for an appointment. (C. Wait until after the meeting with the emergency department physician director and nursing supervisor.)

Now you know the most effective use of your time. You should start calling the other ambulance services in your area to learn how they handle problems with the emergency department and call to make an appointment to meet with the emergency department physician director and the nursing supervisor as soon as possible. After the As are done, move on to the Bs, and finally if time allows, the Cs. Rarely does everything get done.

Learning to say no

Some managers have difficulty saying no to protect their time. Admittedly there are occasions when you really can't say no. For example, you might be interrupted and have to stop working on your A1 if your boss calls and wants to know why the new ambulance costs so much. But those occasions should be the exception and not the rule. In general you must learn to say no if you are to control your time. (We will cover the topic of assertiveness in Chapter 5.)

It's important for you to remember that you can control the timing on virtually all activities that you undertake. Your time is valuable, so you shouldn't allow its control to pass over to others just because they ask you for a minute. Most people won't be hurt if you put them off temporarily. But be sure to schedule them later. They probably would be hurt if you never got back to them.

Avoiding crisis management

Sometimes a crisis will arise, and you will have to stop working on your A1. However, if you are to manage your time wisely, you must first recognize what a real crisis is. Don't get hooked into treating problems as crises just because people are excited or angry. For example, a common problem facing many emergency department nursing supervisors is a physician becoming angry because he has not been called for one of his patients. Often the physician storms into the nursing supervisor's office and demands that something be done immediately. Although it is important that the nursing supervisor effectively handle the physician's anger, the supervisor should not treat problems of this sort as crises just because the physician is angry.

EMS managers should have a perspective on crisis management that managers in other areas do not share. Most know what a real crisis is because they have been EMTs, nurses, or physicians in life-or-death situations. Remember this:

There is no crisis in EMS management as serious as an upper airway obstruction.

It is essential to keep that sense of perspective.

Some services become so bogged down in artificial crises that the manager can do little but bounce from one crisis to another. To avoid this, you must understand four things:

1. Crises are rarely what they initially appear. They are usually caused by people who are trying to force their own way.
2. There is a big difference between an urgent problem and an important problem. You must continually focus on what is important.
3. You should intervene only in those important crises that cannot be delegated or ignored.
4. You can avoid most real crises with adequate planning.

In summary, effective work planning requires you to establish broad goals, then break those goals down systematically into doable activities and daily tasks. You must write these down on a regularly scheduled basis. You need to prioritize each list to ensure that your time is spent as productively as possible.

Make no mistake: There is nothing mystical about this process. If anything, it is characterized by clarity and simplicity. True, you will be forced into a certain degree of regimentation. But think of the potential reward: You can parlay a relatively small investment of time (perhaps half a day every year, 30 minutes once a month, and 10 minutes each day) into a far more effective use of the rest of your time. You use 2 percent of your time to direct the other 98 percent. The alternative is spending 100 percent of your time randomly. If your time schedule is so hectic that you feel that you can't afford to spend 2 percent of it on planning, your need for these time management tools is all the more critical.

Avoiding timewasters

Let's look at some specific activities, called *timewasters*, that cripple your effectiveness as a manager.[6] If you want to use your time optimally, you need to eliminate these timewasters from your day.

To develop this list of timewasters, we asked people providing medical care to list those things that wasted their time. They indentified the following timewasters (listed in order of importance):

1. Interruptions
2. Personal disorganization
3. Procrastination
4. Lack of delegation
5. Meetings
6. Not saying no
7. Lack of persistence
8. Poor communication

These timewasters probably affect you—robbing you of time that you could spend on your life or work goals.

Which timewaster should you work on first? Start by prioritizing the list of timewasters. Your list might look like this:

1. Interruptions—A3
2. Personal disorganization—B

3. Procrastination—C
4. Lack of delegation—A2
5. Meetings—A1
6. Not saying no—B
7. Lack of persistence—C
8. Poor communication—C

Look up your A1 timewaster (meetings) in the timewaster analysis at the end of this chapter. You will find 17 causes of ineffective meetings. Review the list and select those causes that affect you. Perhaps for you the failure to abolish committees when their work is accomplished is the major cause of wasted time. You sit on several committees that are no longer useful. Read the solution from the timewaster analysis: Abolish or quit attending those committees that have outlived their usefulness. Put that activity on your daily to-do list. Do it today and you'll begin saving time.

When you have solved your A1 timewaster, move on to A2. Keep at it. Timewasters are always trying to sneak in.

Summary

To manage effectively in EMS, you must first learn to manage yourself. Understanding your own life goals and how your work fits into those goals is a key to success. Once you have completed that, you can improve your performance as a manager by evaluating your work. Setting work goals and priorities helps you concentrate your attention on those tasks that are most important. Making daily to-do lists plans your workday. Avoiding activities that produce insignificant outcomes and eliminating timewasters ensure that you don't squander your valuable time.

The goal of this chapter has been to put you in control of your life and your work through effective planning. If you've completed this chapter, you have a head start over 90 percent of EMS managers. Your effort to improve your performance as a manager is just beginning, however, because in addition to planning your life and work you must learn and apply planning techniques to your emergency medical service.

Timewaster Analysis 1
INTERRUPTIONS

CAUSE	SOLUTION
1. No plan for handling phone calls.	Have someone screen calls. Set periods for placing and receiving calls.
2. Office door always open.	Recognize that this invites frequent unimportant interruptions. Make sure your staff knows that your door is open for those who need assistance. Close it for periods of work and concentration.
3. Feeling that you must always be available.	Don't overestimate your importance.
4. Desire to be involved in work details.	Routine involvement in detail leads to loss of employee motivation and often wastes your time. Delegate authority and direct people and calls to your subordinates. (See Chapter 7.)
5. Fear of offending others.	Don't be oversensitive. Learn to stand up for your own needs without causing resentment. (See Chapter 5.)
6. Inability to terminate conversations.	Learn and practice: 1. Limit time ("I can talk for a few minutes.") 2. Foreshadow ending (". . . before we finish. . . .") 3. Be candid ("Sorry, I have to go now.")
7. People routinely call you without thinking.	Change number.
8. Beeper.	Have calls screened before you are beeped.
9. Too many calls at home.	Request an unlisted number. Inform coworkers that calls are an unwelcome interruption of your private time.
10. Inability to close door in your location.	Plan time away from office where you'll be unavailable for interruptions.
11. Interrupting others.	Remember, whenever you call or visit someone, you interrupt them. Ask yourself, "Is this call or visit really necessary?"

Timewaster Analysis 2
PERSONAL DISORGANIZATION

CAUSE	SOLUTION
1. Lack of goals, priorities, and daily plan.	Establish goals, priorities, and daily to-do list.
2. Cluttered desk.	Clear desk of everything except what you're working on. Throw out unimportant items. Have a place for everything that is important. Return items to their proper place when finished.
3. Desire to look busy.	Recognize you may also look disorganized, indecisive, insecure, and confused.
4. Failure to delegate.	Delegate anything you can. (See Chapter 7.)
5. Too much paper work.	Handle each piece of paper once. Don't read junk mail. Get off mailing lists. Reply to letters immediately by writing reply on the original letter.
6. No self-discipline.	Impose deadlines on yourself. Try goals, priorities, and daily plan for one month.
7. Procrastination.	See timewaster 3.
9. No secretary.	Minimize paperwork, respond on original. Simplify filing system.
10. Overcommunication.	Emphasize brevity. Don't send out unnecessary paper work and create problems for others.
11. Responding to the urgent.	Distinguish urgent from the truly important. Be more discriminating in sorting priorities.
12. Success without planning.	Recognize success may be *in spite of,* not *because* of, your actions. Planned results are predictably more successful than chance results.
13. Seemingly overwhelming tasks.	Use Swiss cheese technique. Poke holes in your overwhelming tasks by doing a little of the task at a time.
14. Action orientation.	Recognize many problems result from action without thought. So take time to think things through. *Then* act.
15. Unrealistic time estimates.	Recognize that everything takes longer than you think (Murphy's second law).

Timewaster Analysis 3
PROCRASTINATION

CAUSE	SOLUTION
1. No techniques for improving.	Set deadlines on all goals and priorities. Reward yourself when you meet deadlines.
2. No self-imposed deadlines.	Set deadlines on everything.
3. No monitoring of progress.	Have secretary or associate check your progress against deadlines.
4. Uncertain priorities.	Make daily to-do list.
5. Fear of mistakes.	Learn from your mistakes. Don't blame yourself or others.
6. Attempting too much.	Set more realistic goals. See timewaster 2.
7. Unrealistic time estimates.	Recognize everything takes longer than you think. Don't schedule every minute. Leave some time free.
8. Habit.	By adopting good time management techniques, you can break the habit.
9. Doing what you like, postponing the unpleasant. Doing the easy or trivial.	Prioritize your to-do list. Follow the priorities.
10. Overwhelming tasks.	Use Swiss cheese technique. (Poke holes in overwhelming task by doing little bits at a time.)
11. Paper shuffling.	Handle each piece of paper just once.
12. Tendency to put things off.	Remember: "Do it now."

Timewaster Analysis 4
LACK OF DELEGATION

CAUSE	SOLUTION
1. Fear of failure.	Recognize your fear. Learn from mistakes.
2. Lack of confidence in staff.	Train them.
3. Too much involvement in detail.	Keep eye on big picture, not details.
4. Fear of asking employees to do more.	Realize that added responsibility is a prime motivator.
5. Unclear directions.	Have subordinate summarize instructions to you to make sure he has understood.
6. Envy of subordinate's ability.	Realize your envy. If a subordinate is truly talented, you can't keep it from becoming apparent. Use that talent in the organization's best interest.
7. Ability to do job better yourself.	Consider: What is the best use of your time right now? The issue isn't whether you can do the job better. Often you can. If your subordinate can do an *acceptable* job on the task, the best use of your time is to do something else.
8. Enjoyment of "doing."	Realize that your job is *managing*. Most managers are promoted because they were good doers. Doing isn't managing.
9. Poor control.	Don't try to control small details. Look for results.
10. Reverse delegation.	Refuse to make decisions for subordinates if inappropriate.

Timewaster Analysis 5
MEETINGS

CAUSE	SOLUTION
1. Too many meetings.	Attend selectively. Test need for "regular" meetings. Occasionally don't hold them or don't attend and see what happens.
2. Standing committees.	Avoid if possible.
3. Failure to start on time.	If chairman, start on time: if member, speak up. (Delaying for late arrivals penalizes those who arrive on time and rewards those who come late.)
4. Failure to end on time.	If chairman, end on time. Otherwise you make it impossible for participants to plan following meetings. If member, leave on time.
5. Lack of purpose.	Chair or attend no meeting without a purpose and agenda.
6. Wrong people, time, or place.	Select carefully.
7. Socializing.	Reserve socializing for better place.
8. Interruptions.	Set policy and let everyone know. If possible allow no interruptions except for emergencies. Hold calls.
9. Wandering from agenda.	Demand adherence to agenda.
10. Failure to set ending time or time allotments for each subject.	Time-limit the meeting and each item on the agenda.
11. People kept after they are no longer needed.	Leave after expected contribution made.
12. Indecision.	Keep working on issue at hand and its solution.
13. Lack of adequate information.	Collect pertinent information before meeting.
14. No summary.	Summarize conclusions to ensure agreement and remind participants of assignments.
15. No minutes.	Record decisions, assignments, and deadlines in concise minutes.
16. No follow-up.	Make sure commitments are understood and reported at next meeting.
17. Failure to abolish committees when no longer needed.	Stop attending or abolish committee once its business or objectives are accomplished.

Timewaster Analysis 6
INABILITY TO SAY NO

CAUSE	SOLUTION
1. Failure to examine consequences of saying yes.	Remember that saying yes to a meeting or lecture may be saying no to a son or daughter.
2. Lack of excuses.	Realize that you don't need excuses. Sometimes no excuse is better than a poor one.
3. No time to think of answer or excuse.	Take your time and assess the consequences of saying yes. Who says you have to answer immediately?
4. Tradition of organization.	Recognize that many people in the organization probably feel same problem. They may encourage more assertive behavior. Discuss it openly with them. Ask for time management or assertiveness course.
5. Desire to be nice guy.	Understand that if desired results are *not* achieved, you may lose instead of gain respect.
6. Fear of offending.	Develop techniques of saying no without offending. True friends are not offended by honest explanation. (See Chapter 5.)
7. Success.	Recognize this makes you more in demand and makes ability to say no even more important.
8. False sense of obligation.	Understand why you feel that way. Then control it.
9. Insecurity or low self-esteem.	Remember that saying yes will not improve self-esteem. Begin to work on your life goals. Protect your time. As you begin to achieve, self-esteem will increase.
10. Fear of retaliation.	Reassess relationships if person can't accept your saying no.
11. Desire to be productive.	Realize that you can't do everything for everybody.

Timewaster Analysis 7
LACK OF PERSISTENCE

CAUSE	SOLUTION
1. No system for completing tasks.	Use system outlined in this chapter.
2. Responding to the urgent.	Recognize that urgent matters rarely are as important as they seem.
3. Attempt to do too much.	See timewaster 2.
4. Cluttered desk and personal disorganization.	See timewaster 2.
5. Fear of tackling major task.	Poke holes in major tasks (Swiss cheese technique). Break task into small parts.
6. Lack of determination to complete tasks.	Impose deadlines on yourself and let someone else know (committee, secretary, etc.).
7. Inability to delegate.	See timewaster 4 and Chapter 7.
8. Interruptions.	See timewaster 1.
9. Indecision.	Try to understand the cause. (Are you afraid of failure?) Then think it through. How can I reduce the chance of failure?
10. Distraction.	Analyze distractions and eliminate them.

Timewaster Analysis 8
POOR COMMUNICATION

CAUSE	SOLUTION
1. Lack of time.	Take it. Priority warrants.
2. Inattention.	Realize active listening skill must be developed. (See Chapter 5.)
3. Use of wrong method.	Select appropriate method (phone, letter, memo, conference).
4. Poor timing.	Realize that if you select wrong time, the whole message may be lost.
5. Overcommunication.	Don't waste other people's time. Be brief.
6. Undercommunication.	Assess needs for information. Set up regular meeting time if necessary.
7. Lack of policies and procedures for effective communication.	Develop them. Don't ignore informal networks or communications that exist in most organizations.
8. Lack of receptivity.	Test receptivity: "Would you like to talk about . . .?"
9. Poor receptivity.	Recognize that experience, training, and environment create different backgrounds for interpreting communication.
10. Not understood.	Avoid jargon. Talk clearly and concisely.

2

Planning for your EMS organization

The development of our EMS system was chaotic. Of course, I knew nothing about management by objectives. In fact, none of us had any management training. Looking back, I think we were able to accomplish what we wanted to do; but because we weren't well organized, we worked a lot harder than we had to.

—AN EARLY DEVELOPER OF EMS

The time management techniques in Chapter 1 provide you with a systematic way of planning your life and work. As a manager, you must also apply structured management planning to your emergency medical service if your service is to be effective.

Without structured management planning, EMS managers work too hard for too few results. For example, we observed the working of an emergency medical services committee operating in a large city. The local EMS program had many problems, and the committee was working to solve them. The committee held long monthly meetings in which the members complained about the problems with the system. The meetings adjourned with no direction as to who would do what to solve the problems. A month later the committee returned and repeated the whole process. The committee accomplished little, and the EMS problems remained.

In this example several factors limited the committee's effectiveness. For one thing, the meetings were poorly run. For another, committee members didn't listen to one another. But a major reason for failure was the lack of structured management planning to force the committee to move forward toward solving the EMS problems. If you manage in such a situation, you'll waste time, and your service will very likely go nowhere. You need structure.

Many EMS personnel resist formal system planning, often for good reasons. Here's what frequently happens: An EMS manager will feel the need to improve his service's way of planning. He goes away to a management course, where he is taught the "correct" way of applying structured management planning. He returns home armed with new forms, convinced that if his personnel can carefully fill in these forms, his service's planning problems will be over. His personnel resist filling out the forms, and after months of haggling over the system, the manager abandons it. His planning problems remain unsolved.

Why does this happen? There are two reasons:

1. The consultants who teach most management courses usually have little or no practical experience applying structured planning methods to EMS. Consequently they emphasize the "correct" way of applying structured planning methods, rather than teaching how those methods have been applied to EMS.

33

2.   Inexperienced managers often think that the most important part of structured planning is the paper work. All structured planning methods require new forms and paper work. However, cranking out manuals, filling out forms, and setting review dates are meaningless unless they help you to accomplish your goals.

How do you apply structured management planning to EMS? Most planning systems originated in business or in the military. In the early 1970s, alert EMS managers began adapting these systems to emergency medicine. In the decade since then, EMS managers gained considerable experience applying these methods. From this experience, three principles emerge:

1. Different types of EMS organizations have different planning needs.

In this chapter we will introduce you to four basic planning methods: management by objectives (MBO), priority planning (PP), managing for motivation (MFM), and project evaluation and review technique (PERT). Depending on the nature of your service, you'll need to tailor your planning to your needs. You'll need to pick and choose from the methods that we outline in this chapter in order to develop a program that is right for your situation.

2. The simpler the planning system the better.

Groups that attempt to use complex planning methods often run into trouble. Try to keep whatever planning system you use as simple as possible.

3. It takes at least two years to determine whether a planning system will work.

Introducing structured planning into EMS will meet resistance. (We'll cover the topic of resistance to change in Chapter 8.) As a manager, you'll need to manage that resistance effectively. Remember that in the first few months almost all systems appear to be failing. Don't give up during that period. You must work with a planning system at least two years before you can truly evaluate its effectiveness.

Analyzing your current organizational structure

Before you consider what type of planning to introduce into your service, you must evaluate what planning system methods your total organization has. For example, if you manage a municipal ambulance service, check what sort of planning your city government uses. If it uses management by objectives, then it makes sense for you to be consistent and use MBO also.

In many cases you'll find that your organization uses no specific technique. That's what we found when we sought to introduce structured planning into a rural EMS system. A consultant whose aid we enlisted told us that we would very likely fail if we tried to introduce structured management planning into only one part of an organization that used no specific planning technique. He told us that to succeed, we needed to introduce the program into the whole organization. This was the prevailing feeling in the early to mid-1970s, and it prevented some EMS managers from applying structured planning. They questioned, "Why bother applying it to my service if I'm destined to fail because the whole system hasn't adopted a planning system?" In the last few years, however, it has become clear that success in introducing structured management planning methods depends more on your ability to select the correct method and handle resistance to its introduction than it does on the use of the method in the organization as a whole. Often, when structured management planning is successfully applied to one part of an organization, other parts of the organization will adopt it, tailoring it to their particular needs. Structured management planning actually seems to work better when it is introduced in this way, instead of being imposed upon an entire organization from the top.[1]

The four basic planning methods are summarized in Table 2–1, and a discussion of each follows. It's important for you to determine which planning method will work best for your service. You may find that one of the four methods that we outline will work best for you. However, you'll probably select a combination of approaches; certain methods will work best in certain situa-

TABLE 2–1. Management Planning Methods

MANAGEMENT BY OBJECTIVES (MBO)

Key Features: Defines organization's mission and goals. Identifies short-term objectives.

Advantages: Most common planning system. Good for completing tasks where objectives are clear.

Disadvantages: Not particularly helpful for day-to-day running of system. Difficult to use when objectives are unclear.

PRIORITY PLANNING (PP)

Key Features: Divides jobs into key elements; rates key elements against minimally acceptable performance.

Advantages: Assists in keeping track of day-to-day responsibilities. Helps manager to decide what to do next.

Disadvantages: Not well-suited for major tasks. Relies heavily on manager's rating of performance. Some consider paperwork a burden.

MANAGING FOR MOTIVATION (MFM)

Key Features: Uses questionnaire to determine employee motivation. Presents data so that manager can determine problem areas.

Advantages: Helps ensure people are well-motivated. Good for times when services have poorly defined problems or when objectives are unclear. Solicits employee input.

Disadvantages: Needs small computer to work best. Some employees resent questionnaire. Rarely adequate when used alone—usually needs to be combined with another system.

PROJECT EVALUATION AND REVIEW TECHNIQUE (PERT)

Key Features: Uses chart to display activities and events involved in completing a task.

Advantages: Forces manager to plan a task carefully. Best system for planning major projects. Enables the manager to use resources effectively.

Disadvantages: Not helpful for routine tasks or when work objectives are unclear. Usually needs to be combined with another planning system.

tions. Let's start our review with the most common structured planning method, management by objectives.

Management by objectives

Developed by management consultant Peter Drucker, management by objectives has been a major topic of discussion and debate in management circles since the 1960s.[2] We've condensed Drucker's important ideas in this chapter, where we provide you with the basics to put an MBO system in place.

It's important that you understand MBO for two reasons. First, MBO is the most common system that you'll encounter in EMS. Second, other structured management methods are designed to overcome flaws in MBO.

The first step in using MBO is to determine the goals of your service. Drucker tells an old story about three stonecutters who were asked as they worked what they were doing. The first responded, "I am making a living." The second answered, "I am doing the best job of stonecutting in the entire country." The third looked skyward and said, "I am building a cathedral." Obviously the third one thought as a manager should think—he knew how his work fit into the bigger picture of the entire task.[3]

You must think like the third stonecutter. You must determine how your service and its goals fit not only into your total organization but also into the entire field of EMS and the even larger fields of public safety and health care. To do this, you should ask yourself and your personnel, "What are we trying to accomplish here?" In answering this question, you'll gain both ideas and later support for achieving your goals if you seek input from others, both inside and outside your organization. Input from your staff is extremely valuable in identifying specific problems and potentials of your service; after all, who should know your service better than the people who work for it every day? Whether you gain this input from a formal planning committee or through informal discussions with individual employees isn't important. What matters is that you involve your staff in the planning process at the earliest possible time.

In seeking input you must also involve people outside your service. Remember: No matter whether your service is privately owned or part of a larger nonprofit organization, you are still providing emergency medical care to the general public. As such,

TABLE 2–2. Sources of Public Input for Goal Setting

City or county governments
Citizen advisory groups
Hospital boards of trustees
Regional or state EMS councils
Civic organizations (e.g., United Way)
Ambulance service boards of directors

you must gain planning input from the public to determine in which directions to develop your service. Clearly you don't want to expand ambulance service into an area where there is no demand. Your service's success will depend on your ability to match your service's plans to the public's desires for emergency services and their ability to pay for them. Table 2–2 lists six existing groups that EMS managers have used for outside input.

In addition to relying on formal, outside groups for input you may want to consult various individuals informally concerning your service's goals. Try to obtain opinions from a wide range of individuals. Consulting only those individuals who strongly support EMS and your service will give you an unrealistically bright view of the future.

From your discussion with people inside and outside your service you should be able to develop a list of overall goals for your service. In EMS the major goal cited is usually to save lives. Although it may be easy to reach agreement that your major purpose is to save lives, you may have some difficulty reaching a consensus on exactly how you are going to accomplish this. If you manage a nonprofit suburban ambulance service, you might list four goals designed to save lives:

- Provide 24-hour-a-day, competent, advanced-life-support ambulance service to the county.
- Develop cooperative relationships with surrounding ambulance services and the county hospital.
- Develop a fiscally responsible system that does not rely on the continuous infusion of state and federal funds.
- Participate actively in the development of EMS on a county and state level.

In developing this list you must answer several fundamental questions:

- What type of care will we provide?
- At what level are we going to provide care?
- What area will we cover?
- What hours will we be available?
- How are we going to relate to other EMS organizations?
- How are we going to support ourselves financially?

How you answer these questions will have a profound impact on the overall design of your service. At this stage of the MBO process you must resolve differences of opinion on what the system is to become. If, for example, your board of directors thinks that the area can support only a basic-life-support service, but your personnel want to be state-of-the-art, you must try to develop an acceptable compromise. It's important that you hammer out as many of these differences as possible. Don't sidestep issues. They will return to haunt you in the form of lack of cooperation and cohesion.

We call this first step deciding organizational goals. Although this step gives you a clearer picture of where your service is heading, it doesn't ensure that you'll accomplish anything. To do that, you must determine short-term objectives.

Setting objectives

There is no magic time frame for setting objectives; you could use five years, three years, one year, or whatever you like. Yearly objectives work nicely in EMS management for several reasons. First, as a field, EMS changes rapidly. Who knows what will happen in the next year, two years, or five years? Objectives established for time periods longer than one year often lack precision; constant change makes setting practical objectives for longer periods impossible. Second, EMS personnel don't like to deal with a lot of lists. Convincing people to work with yearly objectives is hard enough. If you bury people in constantly changing lists of objectives, MBO becomes more of a problem than it is worth. Third, a year is a good time frame for conducting major projects. You can upgrade an ambulance service to a higher skill level in a year if you hustle. You can design new education programs in a year. Finally, many contracts and budgets run on one-year cycles. It makes sense to have your objectives cover the same period as the money that funds them.

When writing your objectives, follow these guidelines:

ACCEPTANCE. Don't add an item to your service's list of objectives unless it is accepted by a consensus of your service's key people.

MEASURABILITY. Make sure that objectives are measurable so you know if and when you've accomplished them. Don't hide behind objectives like *continue working on new education program*. Transform them into objectives like *complete first draft of course summary*. Start off with an action verb like *complete, train,* or *purchase*.

ACHIEVABILITY. Select objectives that you can actually accomplish. Although some people may find it noble to pursue unattainable objectives, most people become frustrated and burn out when they continually attempt to achieve the impossible.

TIME LIMITATIONS. As we said, yearly objectives often work well in EMS. While it doesn't matter greatly whether you set objectives every six months or every year, it is extremely important that you apply some deadline. People often put off completing objectives when they have no deadline. Of equal importance is the concept of closure. We all need to feel that we have finished a task or are moving toward a goal. We can take pride in our achievement when we are finished. Unless you set some time limitations on your objectives, it will be difficult to stop and tally your results—enjoying what you have been able to achieve.

SIGNIFICANCE. Every emergency medical service has hundreds of objectives. Some are major; most are minor. Don't pad your list of objectives with trivial activities that you can easily complete. Although you may think that this makes you or your service look good, it doesn't. If you have only one or two important objectives for a year, concentrate on accomplishing those. Don't get bogged down in triviality just so that you can look busy.

These rules should guide you in your attempts to write meaningful objectives for your service. Let's return to our example of the suburban ambulance service. Your yearly objectives might be:

1. Train 11 EMTs in ACLS (Advanced Cardiac Life Support).

2. Staff 1 ACLS-trained EMT on each ambulance run.
3. Increase ambulance service volume by 5 percent.
4. Develop a cooperative regional ambulance agreement.
5. Develop a cooperative agreement with a hospital.
6. Institute financial management program.

Note how these yearly objectives follow the previously developed goals. There is no rule that states that in any year your objectives must reflect all your goals. If it makes sense this year that all your objectives reflect only one of your goals, so be it.

Monthly commitments

In EMS it is necessary to divide objectives into small pieces—monthly commitments. Monthly commitments should have all the characteristics of yearly objectives: acceptance, measurability, achievability, time limitations, and significance. The difference is that each key administrative participant should make commitments to reflect how he is going to contribute to fulfilling the service's objectives. Although you needn't necessarily adopt a time frame of one month, we have found that this works well in EMS management for several reasons. First, many EMS systems hold monthly meetings, which provide a convenient opportunity to review commitments. Second, one month is a healthy compromise between feeling burdened with paper work (if commitments are made weekly) and forgetting what you've committed to do (if commitments are made quarterly). Third, month-size bites are an effective way to break apart big tasks. If you select commitments that reflect what you can achieve during the next month, your work will rarely intimidate you. Finally, sharing commitments with your coworkers provides an effective structured communication mechanism. One month seems a practical time frame to keep people up-to-date.

Monthly commitments are important because they link your life and work goals (developed in Chapter 1) with your organizational goals and objectives. Figure 2–1 demonstrates that relationship.

As you learned in Chapter 1, you should prioritize your monthly commitments. The prioritized list then provides the basis for constructing daily to-do lists.

These steps represent the fundamentals of MBO. In MBO you determine what your organization is trying to do, divide that

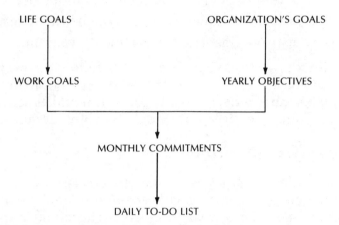

FIGURE 2-1. How Management by Objectives Merges with Manager's Personal Planning

into definable objectives, and break the objectives into smaller commitments. On the surface, MBO seems like a perfect organizing system for EMS. In practice, however, MBO has two major pitfalls:

1. **Emphasis on once-through tasks.** If you examine the yearly objectives for an EMS system, you will see a predominance of once-through tasks, i.e., tasks that you don't do repetitively. Such lists rarely contain things like make sure that the ambulances are in good running shape every day or make sure that we follow protocols on every ACLS case. Instead they emphasize buying a new ambulance or building a new emergency department. If you follow only your MBO yearly objectives, you might accomplish several major items, but the day-to-day running of your service might fall apart.

2. **Unclear objectives.** Drucker himself has written: "Management by objectives works if you know the objectives. Ninety percent of the time, you don't." Consequently in MBO you often concentrate your yearly objectives on the easily identified tasks that you must perform. Unclear

tasks don't lend themselves to a quick listing on your yearly objectives.

Despite these two problems, **MBO** is extremely valuable in **EMS** management. To overcome the deficiencies of **MBO**, you are probably going to use at least part of another planning method.

Priority planning

EMS managers adapted priority planning to emergency medical management in the early 1970s.[4] To build a priority planning system, you first need to determine the areas for which you are responsible, called *key elements*. Suppose that you are an administrator in charge of a large, hospital-based EMS system, which includes an ambulance service, an emergency department, and an intensive care unit. You might identify 17 key elements for your job:

1. Nursing
2. Ambulance service
3. Administration
4. Medical staff
5. ER physicians
6. State EMS
7. Hospitals
8. Public relations
9. Special medical services
10. Quality assurance
11. Meetings
12. Emergency department
13. Education
14. Legal
15. Intensive care
16. EMTs
17. Management systems

These key elements identify your major areas of responsibility.

The second step in priority planning is to divide each area of responsibility into its component parts. You might break down the legal area as follows:

1. Licenses
   a. Physician
   b. Nursing
   c. EMT
   d. Vehicle
2. Policies
   a. Permission to treat
   b. No code
   c. Intoxicated patient
   d. Release of information
   e. Emancipated minor
   f. Rape
   g. Child abuse
3. Relationships
   a. Local law enforcement
   b. District attorney
   c. Local attorneys
   d. Medical examiner
   e. Other ambulance services
4. Special Cases
   a. Workman's compensation
   b. Malpractice
   c. Medical control
5. Forms
   a. Emergency Department record
   b. Ambulance run report form
   c. Refusal of treatment

In priority planning you need to break down all your key elements like this. This process usually results in a list of over a hundred items for which you are routinely responsible.

The key concept behind priority planning is Minimally Acceptable Performance (MAP). The MAP is the level of performance that you as a manager consider minimally adequate to meet the needs of your service. Follow these guidelines in establishing your MAP:

1. Realize that your MAP reflects a particular time. Ask yourself, "What is the minimal performance I expect at

this time?" You'll probably expect future performance to be better, but be careful not to overestimate your current MAP because of those expectations.

2. Don't play favorites. All EMS managers have certain areas that they like better than others. Recognize that to be effective you must ensure adequate performance in all areas of responsibility.

3. Pay attention to details. Because you've already broken down your key elements into lists of smaller items, you know what details are important. At regular intervals you reexamine those lists to review the details of the areas for which you are responsible.

Following these guidelines, you can determine the MAP for each key element and list it on a priority planning profile work sheet. Figure 2–2 shows how you might rate your key elements.

When you complete your work sheet, you can see the areas that are the farthest below your MAP. You should attack the lowest rated areas first. In this example you should initially concentrate on legal problems. After that you should work on problems with emergency physicians and EMTs. The beauty of priority planning is that it prioritizes the problems that you face. This is extremely helpful for a new manager or a manager working in a

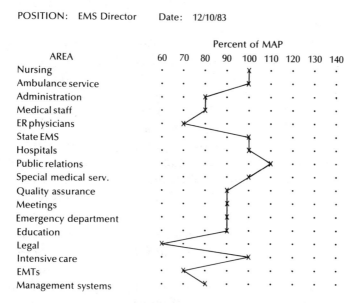

FIGURE 2-2. Priority Planning Profile Work Sheet

service where everything is going wrong. The work sheet doesn't tell you the exact tasks that you need to perform in the lowest rated areas. Through the process of rating your key elements, however, you usually are able to determine what to do.

Priority planning is simple. You divide your responsibilities into areas called *key elements.* At regular intervals you rate the key elements against a minimally acceptable performance standard. You list the ratings on a work sheet. By examining the work sheet you can determine those areas that you need to attack first. Here are some questions that EMS managers frequently ask at this point:

- *How do I determine the performance rates against the MAP in areas like legal or education?* Suppose your problem in the legal area is that you don't have an effective procedure for chain of evidence in rape cases. How much does the lack of that procedure cause your rating of the legal element to be lowered—10 percent, 20 percent? Although you have no clear way of determining this, make the best possible estimate. Ratings are relative. The exact number doesn't matter. What is important is how that number relates to your ratings of other areas. So if the legal element is much worse than education, you might rate legal at 60 percent and education at 90 percent of your MAP.

- *What happens if all of my ratings exceed my MAP?* This is unlikely because most EMS managers are always dissatisfied with something. If all your ratings should exceed your MAP, you can do one of two things. You can raise your standards. If your MAP for your ambulance service were three well-equipped ambulances, you could raise it to four. Alternatively you can leave your standards where they are and attack your least positive area. If the education element is rated at 125 percent of your MAP but is your lowest rated area, concentrate your attention there.

- *When I make my periodic ratings, should I consult my previous rating, or should I determine them blind?* If blind ratings work better for you, use them. Most managers, however, find that consulting previous ratings gives them a greater sense of continuity.

Priority planning solves a major problem of MBO. MBO concentrates on once-through tasks, ignoring for the most part day-to-day responsibilities; priority planning concentrates primarily on day-to-day tasks. Because priority planning requires that you review all the small details that make up your job responsibility, you catch day-to-day mishaps. Priority planning works well when combined with an MBO system. That way, you must pay attention to both day-to-day details and major objectives; as a result, neither managerial responsibility is ignored.

Managing for motivation

Unlike MBO and Priority Planning, Managing for Motivation (MFM) was developed specifically for EMS management.[5] MFM addresses the problems that occur when Priority Planning and MBO are applied to EMS. A major reason why these two systems have difficulties is that the goals of EMS management are more obscure than the goals in other areas of business management. For example, if you are manufacturing widgets, your goal is fairly simple: produce more widgets at a lower cost. You can easily assess the results of your decisions: "We are producing 10 percent more widgets per hour since we redesigned the assembly line."

What are the corresponding goals in EMS? Saving lives is the ultimate goal, but successful cardiopulmonary arrest resuscitations can occur in ineffective, poorly managed services. Money is important, but profitability is not the goal of most services. Utilization is significant, but increased utilization reflects many factors other than performance (e.g., population trends, other health care resources). Patient waiting time, patient complaints, and administrative relations are important, too. Clearly the goals of EMS management reflect a large number of factors.

In the EMS experience MBO works best when objectives are easily defined, and it is very effective in the developmental phase of EMS systems. During development, objectives can be precise; for example, "This year we will train 10 ACLS instructors." However, once EMS systems are in place, the objectives of management can become cloudy.

When objectives are unclear, priority planning is helpful in forcing you to concentrate on the details of your job responsibilities. It enables you to determine which of many deficient areas to attack first. Unfortunately priority planning relies heavily on your perceptions of what is going wrong with your service. As a result, ratings reflect your biases and often your errors.

MFM concentrates on people rather than tasks, focusing on the correlation between employee motivation and job performance. In general, highly motivated employees perform their jobs better than less motivated employees. In EMS, highly motivated employees are often just as important as well-planned tasks. As a result, MFM was designed to enable you to measure employee motivation and plan your service's objectives so that they maximize that motivation.

To understand MFM, you must have some knowledge of employee motivation. There are scores of theories of employee motivation. The two most widely accepted theoreticians are Maslow and Herzberg.[6,7] We will discuss Maslow's theories in Chapter 6. MFM uses Herzberg's theories.

Herzberg and his coworkers interviewed 1,685 employees in 12 investigations to determine what factors affected employee satisfaction and dissatisfaction. These investigations led to the following conclusions:

- Certain job elements, called *hygiene factors,* lead to job dissatisfaction when not adequately present in the work environment. These factors include company policy and administration, supervision, work conditions, and relationships with supervisor and peers.
- Other job elements, called *motivation factors,* lead to job satisfaction when they are adequately present in the work environment. These factors include achievement, recognition, the work itself, responsibility, and advancement.

Like many theories Herzberg's conclusions may be too simplistic. Specifically the distinction between hygiene and motivation factors may not always be clear; some factors affect certain people differently. However, Herzberg's theories are important to EMS because they can be transformed into a useful EMS management tool: managing for motivation. MFM achieves three things:

1. It provides a rapid means of assessing Herzberg's hygiene and motivation factors in the EMS system.
2. It presents data about these factors in a way that the EMS manager can understand and use.

3. It highlights problem areas so that the manager can address them.

MFM assesses motivation factors in the EMS system by means of a questionnaire. Because EMS people don't enjoy paper work, the questionnaire was designed so that it can be filled out in two minutes. A copy of the questionnaire appears on the following page.

The statements in the questionnaire reflect Herzberg's major motivation and hygiene factors. The EMS attitude profile displays the mean scores for the 10 factors for each EMS group. The EMS attitude profile is much like the priority planning profile in that key elements are related to one another so that you can easily see which areas rate the lowest. There are two differences:

1. The attitude profile displays feelings rather than task performance.
2. The attitude profile reflects employees' opinions rather than the manager's opinions.

Figure 2–3 provides an example of how to use MFM.

In the profile in Figure 2–3, four of the five motivation factors for nurses were below 5, meaning that in four of five key motivation areas the nurses responded negatively about their jobs. On the statement on responsibility, 11 of 14 emergency department nurses expressed negative attitudes (scores of 4 or below); the mean score was 3.2. The nurses' responses highlighted a major problem with the design of their work: no one gave the nurses any say in how they did their job.

Before the questionnaire it was clear that many nurses had negative feelings about certain aspects of their jobs. In order to improve this, the EMS manager was spending a great deal of time and effort "helping out" the nurses. What the questionnaire revealed was that this "helping out" was not solving the problem but in fact was part of the problem.

With this information the emergency medical service was able to develop objectives aimed at improving this motivation problem. The nurses selected a new supervisor who delegated authority. The approach to EMS decision making was changed so that nurses participated to a greater degree in determining policies that affected their jobs.

Six months after the first questionnaire the nurses again rated their jobs. This time only 2 of 13 nurses responded negatively to the statement about responsibility; the mean score was

EMS OPINION SURVEY

In order to improve our EMS system, we need to know how you feel about your job. Please fill out this questionnaire. The questionnaire consists of 11 statements. The first is about your job; the other 10 concern your feelings about your job. Please respond to the statements by selecting a number from 1 (strongly disagree) to 9 (strongly agree); 5 means that you neither agree nor disagree.

Example:	Strongly Disagree								Strongly Agree
I like beets	1	②	3	4	5	6	7	8	9

I answered 2. I disagree with the statement. I don't like beets. I never have, despite what my mother says. I didn't answer 1 because I don't hate beets. I hate asparagus. Asparagus would get a 1.

Please be truthful. Your answers are very important. Don't sign the answer sheet. We want all responses to be anonymous. Good luck, and thanks.

1. My current job is (check one)

___ Emergency Department Nurse   ___ EMT or Paramedic   ___ Physician's Assistant
___ Intensive Care Nurse   ___ Secretary   ___ Other
     ___ Physician

	Strongly Disagree								Strongly Agree
2. I get along well with my immediate supervisor.	1	2	3	4	5	6	7	8	9
3. I receive recognition when I do my job well.	1	2	3	4	5	6	7	8	9
4. My job has good prospects for advancement.	1	2	3	4	5	6	7	8	9
5. My working conditions are good.	1	2	3	4	5	6	7	8	9
6. I'm given a lot of say in how I do my job.	1	2	3	4	5	6	7	8	9
7. I agree with department policies as they relate to my job.	1	2	3	4	5	6	7	8	9
8. I enjoy the work I do.	1	2	3	4	5	6	7	8	9
9. I get along well with the people with whom I work.	1	2	3	4	5	6	7	8	9
10. I am well supervised in my job.	1	2	3	4	5	6	7	8	9
11. I feel that I'm achieving a lot in my job.	1	2	3	4	5	6	7	8	9

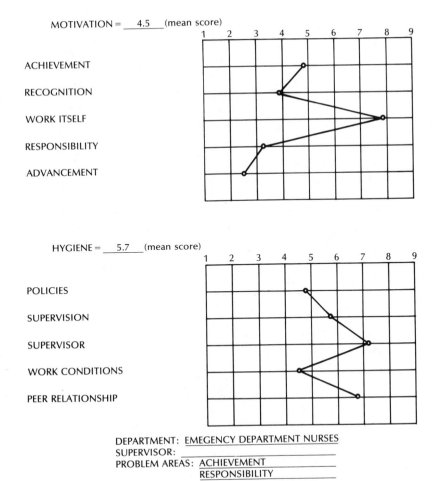

MOTIVATION = __4.5__ (mean score)

ACHIEVEMENT
RECOGNITION
WORK ITSELF
RESPONSIBILITY
ADVANCEMENT

HYGIENE = __5.7__ (mean score)

POLICIES
SUPERVISION
SUPERVISOR
WORK CONDITIONS
PEER RELATIONSHIP

DEPARTMENT: EMEGENCY DEPARTMENT NURSES
SUPERVISOR: _____
PROBLEM AREAS: ACHIEVEMENT
RESPONSIBILITY

FIGURE 2-3. EMS Attitude Profile

6.2. This represented a statistically significant improvement. The objectives developed as a result of the first EMS attitude profile had been successful in dramatically improving motivation.

MFM has several advantages over MBO and priority planning. First, it relies on employee input for determining problem areas. MFM processes that input objectively. As a result, MFM helps eliminate managerial blind spots. Second, all employees provide input to the management system. Often the EMS manager will be close to certain employees and not close to others, or certain employees will be more vocal about their problems. As a result, the manager will have a biased picture of his personnel problems. MFM eliminates this by requiring *all* employees to fill out the attitude questionnaires. Third, when questionnaires are administered at regular intervals, MFM can provide an objective measure of progress in improving the EMS system. Fourth, once MFM defines problems, the manager is forced to return to his employees to determine what they meant when they rated an area low. This often starts a productive dialogue that encourages employee involvement in problem solving.

Like the other systems MFM has its flaws. First, employees often find filling out the questionnaires tedious and resent the intrusion on their time. As a result, you can't circulate the questionnaires more than once every six months or so. Second, MFM works best when a computer is available because the computer can sort the questionnaire information in a variety of ways. Third, MFM doesn't deal with tasks. Consequently MFM must be used with a system like MBO. Fourth, because MFM is new, its long-term effectiveness is uncertain.

Project evaluation and review technique (PERT)

A fourth approach to system planning is project evaluation and review technique (PERT), originally designed for planning large military building projects. EMS managers have used PERT for planning large EMS projects.[8]

The basic operation of PERT is simple. Make a chart on which you identify two major elements:

- **Events.** An event is an identifiable time when an objective is accomplished. In constructing a PERT chart indicate an event by a circle.

- **Activities.** An activity is a task that leads to the completion of an event. Activities begin with one event and end with another. On a PERT chart represent an activity with a line.

PERT charts are a series of circles (events) interconnected with lines (activities). A simple PERT chart would look like Figure 2–4. In this case, activity C connects events A and B. Event A might be sending a check for a cardiac monitor to the manufacturer. Activity C would be the activities that the manufacturer completes in processing your order. Event B would be the arrival of the monitor at your service.

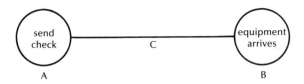

FIGURE 2-4.   Simple PERT Chart

You can place a time estimate on activity C. Your best estimate for the amount of time required for the manufacturer to process your order might be three weeks. So your estimated time of completing this PERT chart would be three weeks.

Some PERT charts contain hundreds of circles and lines. It's easy to be intimidated by a chart like that. But if you remember that PERT charts are always drawn up one circle and one line at a time, you'll find them less frightening.

Let's look at a slightly more complex PERT chart. Suppose that your regional EMS council is trying to negotiate with the local hospitals and ambulance services on a policy for transferring patients. A part of your PERT chart might look like Figure 2–5. In this PERT chart the regional EMS council meets and decides on a tentative agreement. Representatives of the EMS council then meet separately with representatives of the hospitals and the ambulance services. After both meetings are held, the regional EMS council meets again.

The first thing to note about this chart is that it branches after the first EMS meeting. Both the meeting with the ambulance services and the meeting with the hospitals must occur before the second EMS meeting, but they can occur independently of one another; that is, the hospital meeting can occur before or after the

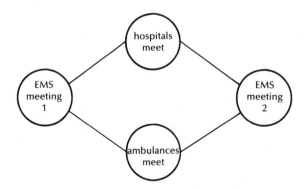

FIGURE 2-5.   Part of a Complex PERT Chart

ambulance meeting. As a manager, this knowledge can help you in planning your efforts. You don't have to wait for one meeting to occur before you begin working on the other.

How long will it take you to complete this chart? Suppose that it's easy to set up the ambulance meeting; you could hold it an hour after the regional EMS meeting. Once the ambulance meeting is completed, it would take you about a week to have the minutes of that meeting ready for the second EMS meeting. On the other hand it will be three weeks before all the hospital participants can meet. It will take you another week to have the minutes of that meeting ready for the second regional EMS meeting. So it will take you a total of four weeks to complete the top path. During those four weeks you'll easily complete the bottom path, which takes only one week. Completing the entire chart will take four weeks. In cases like this, when your PERT chart branches, the pathway that takes the longest time to complete is called the *critical path*. The critical path determines how long it will take you to complete the project.

The critical path determines whether you'll be able to complete tasks by their target date. In this example you should have no problem if you can hold the second EMS meeting in four weeks or more, because it takes four weeks to complete the critical path. However, if you must reach final agreement in three weeks, you definitely have a problem. The time required to complete your critical pathway exceeds the time requirements of your deadline. When this occurs, you must either change your deadline, if possible, or replan the task. In this case, if you had a firm three-week deadline, you could either try to call an urgent meeting of the hospital administrators or hold the second EMS meeting immediately after the hospital meeting, dispensing with typed minutes of the hospital meeting.

This example represents only a small part of a major task, in which your critical path will have scores of events. In major tasks you'll have to make many planning decisions to meet your deadline. In these cases the great advantage of PERT is that you know these things *before* you ever start a project. You know which events must occur precisely on schedule for the program to meet its deadline and which events can be delayed. In this case, for example, you could delay the ambulance meeting for a week without any significant effects. The ability to make decisions like this before the project starts will make your projects run more smoothly. You'll complete more of the tasks that you attempt, and you'll complete them on time.

Pulling the systems together

Remember: Every service and project has its individual needs. You must tailor whatever planning method you use to the problems that you're facing. For many EMS managers the following general approach works well:

1. **Install the basics of an MBO system.** You must give your service some direction. You can do this by asking the fundamental questions necessary for MBO. How do we fit within the larger picture? What are we trying to do? How should we go about it? You should establish yearly objectives and monthly commitments. Experiment with these time frames to ensure that they meet your needs.

2. **Evaluate your needs for improved day-to-day planning.** If you or your fellow managers are unclear about your areas of responsibility or about your current priorities for improving the day-to-day operation of your service, set up a priority planning system. The process of defining key elements and minimally acceptable performance is helpful even if you don't use the entire system. If you are new to a service or if your service is in serious trouble, consider a full-blown priority planning system until you straighten out things.

3. **Determine whether you have motivation problems.** In EMS you need motivated personnel. If you have personnel problems that you can't identify, consider using the managing for motivation (MFM) system. Sometimes you will have to administer the questionnaire only once to understand the nature of the motivation problems you face. Alternatively you may want to administer the questionnaire every six months or every year to catch potential motivation problems before they mushroom into crises.

4. **Use PERT to plan major tasks.** If you face major tasks, PERT will help you. You don't always need to bother with determining the critical path, because major projects don't always have fixed deadlines. The process of determining the types and order of events that you need to accomplish, however, can give you considerable insight into completing the task.

Designing a structured management planning meeting

Many EMS management meetings are ineffective and waste your time. By incorporating structured planning methods into your EMS meetings, you can turn ineffective meetings into power-houses. Here's a basic approach that has been used in many EMS settings since the 1970s.

1. **Review of monthly commitments.** Each participant should review the commitments that he made the previous month and his efforts in completing them. He should then present his commitments for the following month. This informs each EMS manager of what everyone else is doing. It encourages each manager to complete his commitments through peer pressure and provides an opportunity for managers to provide encouragement and advice to one another. In large and complex services this monthly exchange may be the only time when all the members of the EMS management team see where the service is headed.

2. **Review of EMS status.** The second section of the meeting allows one participant, usually the EMS director, to review the status of the service. This review might include a quarterly review of the year's objectives so that each member can see the service's progress, a semiannual review of EMS attitude profiles so that each member can see where his particular area stands relative to the whole group, or a review of progress on any project's PERT chart.

3. **Open discussion.** Once monthly commitments and yearly objectives have been reviewed, the meeting can open up into discussion of major controversial issues where group consensus is important. Participants can also use this part of the meeting for brief announcements that they feel need to be brought to the group's attention.

4. **Summary.** To conclude, each participant in this meeting should share his thoughts on the best and worst aspects of the meeting. This provides a final opportunity for participants to vent problems or to offer suggestions for improving the meeting. Usually this summary generates

positive reinforcement with participants stating, "This is the best meeting I attend" or "I can't believe all the things we get done here."

These four steps can create productive EMS meetings. They reinforce the structured management system and require every member of the EMS management team to participate.

Summary

This chapter provides you with the basics of structured management planning. As an EMS manager, you must apply the proper planning methods to your service if you are to be successful. As you've seen, effective planning for your service meshes with the techniques for planning your life and work described in Chapter 1. Planning is the first essential component of management. Once you complete these planning steps, you can move forward to make your plans reality. The next step in that process is organizing your service's personnel and finances, which we cover in Section II.

II

ORGANIZING

This second section covers managerial organizing skills. It contains two chapters. Chapter 3, "Organizing Your Personnel," covers the techniques that enable you to use your personnel most effectively to meet your goals.

Chapter 4, "Organizing Finances," reviews how you organize your material resources to meet your goals. We'll discuss money and show you how to develop budgets.

3

Organizing your personnel

My biggest problem is my personnel. I spend an inordinate amount of time smoothing out the relations between personnel of different services and different levels within my service. Some of my people just don't seem to understand what it takes to run an operation like this and how they fit into the plan.

—EMT, DIRECTOR OF AMBULANCE SERVICE

Planners are dreamers. They look into the future to see what lies there. In the first section of this book you learned to plan effectively. The techniques that you learned put you ahead of 90 percent of EMS managers. But even when you plan effectively, all you end up with is words on paper. By themselves those words are worth nothing. In this chapter and the next you'll learn how to translate those words into action by organizing your personnel and your finances.

When you organize in EMS, you need to consider three areas:

1. How does my emergency medical service fit into the larger EMS system?
2. How is my emergency medical service organized?
3. How do individual jobs fit within my service? How many and what types of people will I need to fill those jobs?

EMS system organization

Your emergency medical service fulfills a role within a larger emergency medical service system. EMS systems combine the efforts of separate emergency medical services to meet a specific public need: the provision of prompt and competent emergency care.

Governmental agencies usually direct EMS systems, but systems vary widely. You'll need to understand the capabilities and organization of the EMS system to which your service belongs so that you can effectively complete your service's objectives. Figure 3–1 illustrates the design of one type of system. In this figure the state EMS office has a legislated responsibility for coordinating the provision of EMS. The state office then supervises regional EMS councils that direct emergency medical care within regions. Each regional council consists of representatives from each ambulance service, rescue squad, and hospital within the region.

As a first step in organizing your personnel, you must understand how your EMS system is designed. If you have a governmental office responsible for EMS in your area, contact it. It should be able to help you understand how the system is set up.

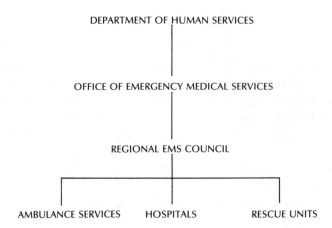

FIGURE 3-1. **Example of EMS System Organization**

Specifically you want answers to the following types of questions:

- **Licensing.** Who has the authority to license and delicense personnel and services? How is it done? Whoever can license and delicense has a great deal of power in the system. How does that agency act? How does it determine if skills are up-to-date? Does it handle skill maintenance training or do you?

- **Medical direction.** Who directs medical care? You need to know how standards of care for your system are developed. If you have regional advanced life support protocols, for example, who writes them? You also need to know what emergency departments operate as base stations for communications. Does one hospital direct all the emergency prehospital care or is that responsibility shared?

- **Cooperation.** How do services cooperate? If you direct an ambulance service, for example, you need to know whether you are solely responsible for covering a geographic area or whether you share that responsibility with others. If that responsibility is shared, how is it done? Do you have mutual aid agreements? If you run a basic-life-support ambulance service, who assists you when you need advanced life support? If you direct an emergency department, what do you do when you're overwhelmed with patients? Do other emergency departments help you? To what hospital do serious trauma patients go?

- **Quality assurance.** Who is responsible for assuring quality? Although each service individually has a responsibility to provide care to the best of its ability, most cases of patient care will involve more than one service. Who is responsible for studying your system's cases to determine whether care is appropriately provided? Some systems have a medical director who fulfills this role. Others have a quality assurance committee. Who studies care for your system and what can that person or group do when a problem is found?

- **Disputes.** Who handles disputes between services? In an emotionally charged field like EMS, disputes between services will occur. Does your system have a committee that settles such disputes? What are its procedures?

You'll need to ask these questions to understand how your system works. Information about your system is crucial in organizing your service effectively. Here's why:

- Suppose that you run a small ambulance service. If you share responsibility for covering a certain geographical area with two other services, you'll probably need fewer personnel than if you had sole coverage, where you need adequate personnel and vehicles to be able to handle almost any possible emergency. If you share coverage, services can cooperate to handle unexpected peak use periods by pooling their personnel and vehicles.

- Suppose that you manage an emergency department with a full-time physician staff. If your system has a paid medical director, you won't have to allocate a portion of one of your physician's time to medical direction activities. This will save you some money and avoid duplication.

- Suppose that you run a volunteer ambulance service and find maintenance of your personnel's skill levels difficult. If the agency that handles licensing your personnel also handles the training for skill maintenance, you won't have to use your limited resources to duplicate their efforts.

By studying your system and the services that it provides, you can save money by avoiding unnecessary duplication. But don't expect your EMS system to be flawless. EMS systems are often political entities, composed of groups looking out for their own needs. As a result you may become somewhat disillusioned when you examine your EMS system. You may find

- Services competing instead of cooperating,
- Personnel with inflated egos standing in the way of progress, and
- Political issues getting in the way of medical care.

Despite the fact that your EMS system may not be ideal, you must understand it and work with it if you are to manage effectively. In Section III you'll learn negotiating and assertiveness skills that will improve your abilities to interact within your system.

Organizing your service

Unless you are a very high offical in EMS, you probably have little impact on how your EMS system is organized. Your own emergency medical service is a different matter. As an EMS manager, you must organize your service's personnel in the most effective manner to meet your service's objectives.

In order to organize your service, you'll have to draw an organizational chart. Figure 3–2 depicts an organizational chart for a private ambulance service.

How do you determine the best organizational chart for your service? There is probably no "best" way. You can organize your personnel in an infinite variety of ways; many of them may be equally effective in achieving your goals. Even among organizational theorists, there is considerable disagreement about many of the basic principles of organization. You don't have time to wade through all the controversies in organizational theory. Let's pick out the key organizational principles and see how they apply to EMS.[1,2]

The work of each person should be confined to a single function.

In general people perform better when they specialize. In EMS, for example, EMTs will perform better if they don't have to do

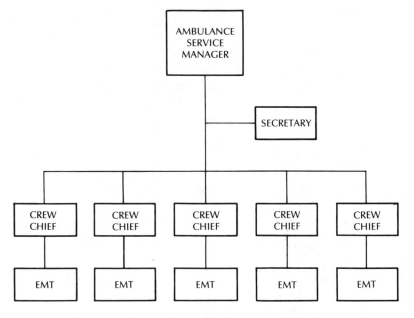

FIGURE 3-2. Organizational Chart for a Private Ambulance Service

secretarial work. Emergency physicans will perform better if they specialize in emergency medicine, rather than if they moonlight in the emergency department. If possible, when you organize your personnel, you should follow this rule. Unfortunately this is not always possible, particularly for small emergency medical services. If you run a two-man ambulance service, you and your partner must be jacks-of-all-trades.

Employees performing related functions should be grouped together.

There are two methods of grouping employees by function: grouping by purpose or by skill. Grouping by purpose is the most common form of organization. The organizational chart of a hospital EMS department in Figure 3–3 illustrates grouping by purpose.

In Figure 3–3 the work force reporting to the EMS director is divided into two sections relating to two specific purposes: (1) the provision of ambulance services and (2) the provision of emergency department services. Each division is a separate entity and fully staffed to meet its goals.

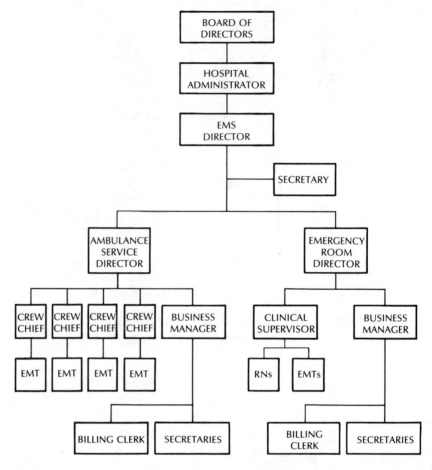

FIGURE 3-3.   Grouping by Purpose

Grouping by purpose has certain advantages: It reduces the dependency of one group on another, it encourages group identity, and it focuses the attention of the group on its specific work goals. There are also disadvantages: Each group may work for its goals at the expense of the service as a whole, cooperation between groups may be lacking, and staffing may be unnecessarily duplicated. In the EMS example in Figure 3-3, separating the emergency department from the ambulance service fosters group identity and working toward group goals, but it may unnecessarily increase staffing and create poor cooperation between EMTs and nurses.

Grouping by skill level is different than grouping by purpose. Figure 3-4 illustrates the same hospital-based EMS service

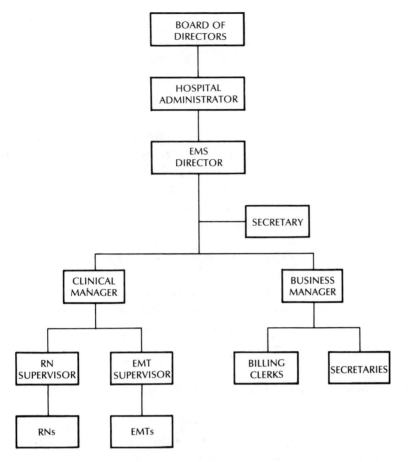

FIGURE 3-4. Grouping by Skill Level

grouped by skill. Grouping by skill level obscures group identity and can limit working toward group goals. On the other hand it can reduce issues of turf. Nurses can move to the ambulance and EMTs to the emergency department. As a result, staffing levels may become more efficient and more flexible. And because group identity becomes less important, service goals transcend group goals.

Each employee in the organization should be accountable to only one superior.

For your service to work well, each employee must have clear direction. That's best accomplished by having each employee accountable to only one supervisor. When an employee is account-

69

able to more than one supervisor, he may become caught in a cross fire of opposite orders. In such cases employees become unproductive and undergo unnecessary stress.

Each supervisor should direct no more than 10 employees.

This rule is not etched in stone. EMS managers have successfully supervised more than 10 employees. In general, however, as the size of your work force increases, you'll face increasing demands in terms of coordinating your service's activities. Suppose, for example, that you manage a successful, expanding ambulance service. It began with 5 EMTs and now has 20. As the number of employees grow, the amount of time that you can spend with each decreases. Monitoring each employee's work becomes more difficult. You can burn out while your employees become dissatisfied with your leadership. In this case you'd probably be much better off if you selected two assistant supervisors from your personnel. You could supervise them and they in turn could supervise 9 EMTs each.

The chain of command should be as short as possible.

This principle puts some limits on the number of levels of supervision. Although you don't want to be the direct supervisor of too many employees, it's also important that you don't have too many supervisors in your chain of command. That would put too many levels of supervision between you and your service's actual work.

If you apply these principles to your service, you should be able to develop a meaningful organizational chart that efficiently utilizes your personnel.

How do jobs fit within your service?

Once you've developed the organizational chart for your service, you need to determine how each job fits within your service. That requires that you write meaningful job descriptions, determine how many positions you need, and train your personnel.

Writing job descriptions

We asked the head nurse in a busy urban emergency department for the department's job descriptions. She pulled a dusty notebook off her shelf and showed us the department's never-used and hopelessly out-of-date job descriptions. A job description should be a useful, up-to-date, detailed written statement that highlights the specific duties and responsibilities that the employee occupying the job should be performing. In EMS, job descriptions like that are rare. If you're like most EMS managers, you dislike the subject of job descriptions. Sitting down to write a job description seems a waste of time. You'd rather be seeing patients or rushing to the scene of an accident. As a result you've probably hastily thrown together job descriptions for your staff, if you've written them at all.

The sooner you reconsider your feelings toward job descriptions, the more effective you'll be. There are three reasons for this:

1. **Writing job descriptions requires that you seriously think about the duties and standards that you expect of your staff.** As a manager, you must organize your personnel so as to accomplish your services's objectives. If you don't take the time to organize your staff, your employees will squander their energies in activities that have little or no bearing on the results that you desire.

2. **Determining proper duties and standards and communicating them with your staff lets each employee know exactly what is expected.** Vague job expectations are a major cause of work-related stress. Your failure to specify exactly what you expect of people can make the already stressful field of EMS even worse for your employees. If you care about your personnel, you'll make job expectations clear. When job expectations are ill-defined, performance falters. People rarely complete poorly understood tasks.

3. **Job descriptions can help you appraise your employees' performance.** How can you fairly say whether an employee is doing a job if you haven't made your job expectations clear in the first place? Well-written job descriptions can be a bench mark for measuring how well your employees complete their jobs. We'll discuss this in greater depth in Chapter 9.

Analyzing the Job

Don't feel bad if your current job descriptions are poor or nonexistent. That's the way it is for many EMS managers. We designed this book to help you escape the traps that catch many EMS managers. A collection of poor job descriptions is one of them.

How do you go about generating useful job descriptions? Many managers have difficulty determining what should go into a job description. If this sounds like you, answer the following questions:

- *What key activities can I identify that should be addressed by this job?* In answering this question you must review your service's goals and determine how this job fits into them. When you drew your organizational chart, you assumed that the person occupying this job would fulfill certain functions that would enable your service to meet its goals. What are those functions?

- *What can I reasonably expect for results and how will they be measured?* In answering this question you will establish performance objectives, which will help you later in the process of performance appraisal. Performance objectives should be specific, measurable, and of a definite time frame.

- *To achieve these results, what will the person have to do?* This question helps you zero in on the specific duties of the job. In answering this question, you begin to examine some of the more structure-oriented parts of the job, such as what the person is responsible for and whom the person supervises.

- *What education and experience would be relevant and helpful in achieving success in this job?* Stressing the *relevance* of education and experience ensures that the hiring process doesn't arbitrarily screen out more people than necessary. You can usually avoid the mistake of asking for unnecessary qualifications by clearly understanding what problems the person should be able to solve.

- *What specific abilities are necessary for this job?* Some people work well under pressure and are easily bored with jobs that are relatively routine. Other people have a low tolerance for stress and can't handle many different problems occurring at once. Some positions require great public-speaking abilities, while other jobs require advanced writing skills. These are all special abilities. As you develop the job description, you should identify as many of these as possible.

Writing better job descriptions

You should consider each of these questions when you establish job descriptions. In addition, your job descriptions will be better if you follow these seven steps:

1. Each job should have a title that is descriptive of the nature and level of the work being performed. Avoid titles that the employee may find objectionable, such as *unskilled EMS clerk.*

2. Begin the description with a general summary. This should state the general nature, level, and purpose of the job. This should be no longer than four sentences. A job summary for an EMT might say: "Provides prehospital assessment, treatment, and transportation for ill and injured patients. Works under the administrative direction of a shift supervisor and the medical director of regional medical control."

3. List the relevant job duties and personal qualities. Describe each one briefly, beginning each sentence with a verb in the present tense. Tell what is done and add an example if necessary. Arrange duties logically and include all tasks that occupy more than 5 percent of the employee's time or are critical to successful performance of the job. Some of the job duties for an EMT might be:

    a. Extricates patients from entrapment.
    b. Assesses the extent of illness or injury in patients.
    c. Identifies diagnostic signs that may require radio communication with a medical facility.

    Personal qualities might include elements such as safety, hygiene, and dependability. Include in this section a summary statement that identifies the job description as a general statement rather than an exhaustive list of all duties for which the employee is responsible. The final EMT job duty might state: "Assists with the func-

73

tional operations of the ambulance service." This reserves your right to request additional duties of the employee later. (Of course, if these new responsibilities involve increased levels of experience, education, or other qualities that affect compensation levels in your service, you may have to regrade the job description to ensure that the employee is being fairly paid. We'll discuss job grading in Chapter 4.)

4. In many cases, particularly where employees perform job duties beyond the routine level, it is helpful to identify within the job description the decision making authority granted to the employee. For example, you might state a dollar limit on expenditures related to decisions which the employee is allowed to make. We'll discuss decision making authority further in Chapter 7.

5. Specify the education and experience levels required to perform the job properly. This will simplify the job grading process later.

6. Describe the working hours and conditions of the job. Remember to include if the job may require unusual hours from time to time. Working conditions should refer both to the physical environment and the physical nature of the job.

7. Identify those employees, if any, who fall under this individual's supervision. Also identify to whom this individual reports.

Establishing job standards

You should include job standards in your job descriptions. A job standard tells exactly how well you expect the job to be done. For example, a paramedic's job performance will meet standard when he "provides prehospital care consistent with protocols and medical control direction 100 percent of the time." List as many job standards for each job duty and personal quality as you need to indicate clearly the level of productivity that you expect. Be sure that each of these performance expectations is within the control of the employee.

The best way to arrive at a standard is by completing the following statement for each duty: *"Performance will be up to standard when...."* In completing this statement, emphasize

TABLE 3-1. Common EMS Job Standards

AREA	STANDARD
Quality	Error rates (tests, medications, X-rays)
	Percentage of work redone
	Percentage of unproductive time
	Number of complaints
Quantity	Number of patients seen
	Number of tasks completed
	Number of ambulance runs
Time	Number of days to complete tasks
	Percentage of tasks completed within time frame
	Number of minutes before a patient is seen
Cost	Percentage variance from budget
	Dollars over a budgeted expense level
	Dollars saved over a previous period

quality, quantity, time, and cost considerations. Table 3-1 illustrates some of the factors that you can assess in these areas.

You can incorporate several of these elements from Table 3-1 into a single standard if appropriate. Suppose, for example, that the job duty for an EMS secretary states: "Prepares weekly reports on the number and type of patients treated." Your standard for how well you want the job performed might state: "With no more than 1 percent error, by Monday of the week following the reporting period."

Once you have completed a job description with job standards, *discuss it with each employee to make absolutely certain that he understands and agrees to work towards it.* Once this process is complete, you have an excellent tool to aid your future assessment of employees' performance during the appraisal process.

Keeping job descriptions current

A job description, once written, isn't accurate forever. EMS goals change over time; as such, your job descriptions must change also. How often should you review your job descriptions? Ideally this exercise should follow your reevaluation of your service's goals; if you reestablish your work goals every year, for example, you might likewise review your job descriptions every year. In any event a year is probably the longest you should go between reviews. You should review job descriptions more frequently if your goals change frequently. If possible, involve the employee in this process to review the job description for accuracy and completeness; this ensures that you and the employee are seeing eye-to-eye on the requirements of the job.

It usually pays to review a job description on an employee's termination. For one thing you may have tailored a job description to a particular individual over time if that employee proved capable of handling increased responsibility. In hiring a new individual you may want to return to the basics of the original job description. You can always add the extra responsibilities if and when you decide the new employee is capable of handling them.

Given the current financial status of EMS, with available dollars shrinking every year, the termination of an employee also provides you with an opportunity to reassess your needs for the position in question; if, for some reason, you find yourself able to meet your needs without this position, it is far easier not to refill the job than to terminate a replacement employee involuntarily later. For these reasons, when a termination occurs you should review the job description, asking yourself a series of questions in the process:

1. *Do the needs that I perceive require a replacement?* If, for example, the job serves to solve a problem that occurs only on an infrequent basis, you may be able to shift someone else's responsibilities temporarily during these periods rather than hiring a permanent, full-time employee.

2. *Can the job be performed successfully by anyone under our present structure?* If, for example, three different people have been hired for the job but quit shortly thereafter in the past year, it's probably time to reanalyze both the job and its place in the organization to see if structural changes in your service are in order.

3. *Can I use an outside service at a lower cost?* If you are uncertain about the long-term nature of your needs in a particular area, you may be further ahead to seek the services of an outside consultant or agency. This can save recruiting, training, and termination costs if your needs prove to be short-lived.

Determining how many positions you'll need

Once you've written effective job descriptions, you must calculate how many positions you'll need. In EMS this is routinely done by examining three factors: coverage, physical limitations, and the amount of work.

Coverage

One characteristic of EMS that is not shared by many other businesses is the concept of coverage. If you run a health clinic, for example, you don't routinely keep the clinic open during hours when you have no patients. That isn't cost-effective. In EMS, on the other hand, you often must staff your service for the possibility that you'll be needed, even if you know that possibility is low.

Suppose that you run a basic-life-support ambulance service, have one ambulance, and are under contract to provide ambulance service coverage to your local community 24 hours a day. If you staff your ambulance with two EMTs, then you'll need two EMTs on duty 24 hours a day.

Coverage is a fairly simple idea. Often in EMS it's the only factor that you must consider in determining the number of positions that you need. Even when you must consider other factors, such as the amount of work performed, coverage generally will determine the minimum number of positions that you need at any one time. You may need more personnel if you have a great deal of work, but you can't have less.

Physical limitations

Certain structural limitations in EMS will determine the maximum number of personnel whom you can have working at any one time. For example, if you routinely staff your ambulance with two EMTs and you have only one ambulance, then the maximum number of positions at any one time is two. If you own two ambulances, it's four. If you run an emergency department that has four patient rooms, the maximum number of nurses whom you can probably use in that physical setup is five—one for each room and one to triage patients. After that the nurses will probably run into each other.

77

There may be times in EMS when you could use more personnel. For example, if you have only one ambulance and receive
two calls at the same time, you'll have more work than you can
handle. If this becomes a constant problem, you may want to consider buying another ambulance. But until you increase your
physical limitations (e.g., buy another ambulance or add rooms
to your emergency department), increasing your staff will not
enable you to do more work.

Work

In EMS, coverage will determine the minimum number of personnel at any one time; physical limitations will determine the
maximum. If your minimum and maximum are the same, such as
in the case of 24-hour coverage with one ambulance, then you
don't need to bother measuring work. If, however, your minimum and maximum are different, then you'll need to determine
appropriate staffing by measuring work.

Work measurement begins by your defining a unit of work.[3]
In EMS this is usually one ambulance run or one patient visit. To
perform work measurement, you must complete four major
steps:

1. Observe and describe the characteristics of a unit of
   work.
2. Estimate the time required to complete a unit of work.
3. Determine the number of units of work that occur during a time period.
4. Determine the number and type of personnel that you
   need to complete those units of work.

Imagine that one of your responsibilities as an EMS manager is
the emergency department. You wish to determine your registered nurse staffing level. Here's how you perform work measurement:

1. You must determine what tasks a nurse performs in
   treating patients. Although you can determine this by interviewing your employees, it's better to observe the
   work directly. What you want to learn is whether the
   nurse is completing tasks that only that individual (or a
   higher skilled person) can do and whether those tasks
   are necessary.

2. Based on your determination of the tasks that a nurse must perform, you should estimate the amount of the nurse's time required for each patient visit. You can also have your nursing personnel fill in survey forms on the time required to treat a group of patients to determine whether your time estimate is correct. Let's say that you determined that an average patient visit requires 20 minutes of nursing time.

3. You review your statistics on patient visits to the emergency department. Review as much data as necessary to give you an accurate estimate of the average number of patients seen each hour, 24 hours a day. That information might look like Table 3–2. You can see that the number of patients ranges from 0.2 to 5.6 per hour.

4. You convert the number of patients into nursing time by multiplying the patient visits times 0.33 hour/visit. This final figure is the number of RNs whom you need in the emergency department per hour on an average day.

"That's all fine," you might be thinking, "but if I staff for an average day, then 50 percent of the time we'll be understaffed." The key to handling this is to adjust the figures that you calculated for patient visits per hour in step 3. If you never want to

TABLE 3–2. Average Number of Patients by Hour Segment

A.M.		P.M.	
Hour Segment	Average Number of Patients	Hour Segment	Average Number of Patients
12 mid.	0.3	12 noon	3.4
1:00	0.3	1:00	4.5
2:00	0.2	2:00	3.8
3:00	0.2	3:00	3.6
4:00	0.2	4:00	3.1
5:00	0.5	5:00	3.0
6:00	0.9	6:00	2.8
7:00	1.8	7:00	2.9
8:00	3.9	8:00	1.7
9:00	5.6	9:00	1.1
10:00	5.0	10:00	1.0
11:00	4.2	11:00	0.7

be understaffed, you could use the maximum visits that your service ever experienced during an hour segment and determine your staffing pattern from that. To be maximally staffed at all times, however, is quite expensive. Generally what you need to do is select a number between the average and maximum staffing that will cover most, but not all, of your busy days. If you have access to a computer, you can do this easily. You put your data of patient visits into the computer and have the computer plot a distribution of how many visits your service experiences. Assuming this approximates a bell-shaped curve (a statistically "normal" distribution), you can have the computer determine mean and standard deviation values. For the information in Table 3–2 for 10 to 11 a.m. the mean value might be 5 and the standard deviation 1. From this information you know that if you staff for five patients, you'll be adequately staffed 50 percent of the time. If you staff for six (one standard deviation above the mean), you'll be adequately staffed about 84 percent of the time. And if you staff for seven patients (two standard deviations above the mean), your staffing will be adequate about 97 percent of the time.

You must realize that in staffing for EMS, you'll never be adequately staffed for everything that might happen. If a 747 crashes on Main Street, you'll be overwhelmed. That's why we have regional disaster plans.

You should also remember that if the staffing levels that you calculated by work measurement exceed your service's physical limitations, then you can't staff at that level. As we said, when your work exceeds your service's physical limitations, there's no point in increasing your staffing until you've increased the physical limitations.

Don't expect perfect results from work measurement the first time you use it. Recognize that your estimates of staffing needs must remain somewhat flexible once you actually implement your staffing system, because real-world factors that you either ignored or misestimated will quickly appear. An entire profession (industrial engineering) exists to perform studies in work measurement, and you can hire these professionals to produce such a study for your service if you want to spend the money. You'll find that you learn a great deal about your service, however, if you try work measurement yourself. You'll also avoid antagonism among your staff if you don't bring in outsiders who "don't understand our operation." Work measurement often spurs controversy because employees dislike monitoring of their productivity. In the long run, however, you will find that the majority of your staff prefers to work in an efficiently run service where workload and staffing levels are properly balanced.

Determining how many people you'll need

By this point you've analyzed the workload of your service to determine the types and numbers of positions that you need to achieve your service's objectives. As a final step you must determine how many people you need to fill those positions. You must do this because your employees don't work 7 days a week, 365 days a year. Your staff needs time off, educational leave, and sick leave. If you determine your staffing levels without thinking about these considerations, you'll underestimate the number of people whom you really need and overwork your staff.

To determine your staffing levels, you must multiply your number of positions by a factor that will yield the number of full-time equivalents (FTEs) that you need. An FTE represents the number of hours of work that you would expect from a routine full-time employee. You determine the multiplier factor by dividing the total number of hours per year that you need a position by the total number of hours per year a full-time employee actually works. In EMS a multiplier of 1.5 is commonly used. Therefore, if you have 4 EMT positions on a 3 p.m. to 11 p.m. shift, you'll need 6.0 people to fill them.

Training your personnel

After you've completed writing your job descriptions and determined how many personnel you need to fill those positions, you must ensure that your personnel possess the skills necessary to meet the standards that you've outlined. No matter how carefully you've applied the lessons that you've learned about personnel organization up to this point, you'll find that your service will fail if your personnel are not adequately trained to meet the standards that you expect of them. To ensure that your personnel are adequately trained, you must understand both the nature of adult learning in general and also what we have found in the 1970s, when adult learning concepts have been applied to EMS situations.

Adult learners

As adults, your personnel enter the educational process with different expectations and needs than do younger people. Consequently the programs that you design and implement for your personnel must be fundamentally different from the learning experience in elementary school, high school, or college. What characteristics of adult learners force this different outlook?[4,5]

1. **Adults have more life experiences.** Because of their experience adults are less likely to accept dogma without questioning it. They are likely to suggest different approaches or concepts. In planning education and training you must respect this experience.

2. **Adults are highly motivated to learn.** Motivation is a key ingredient in learning, and EMS personnel tend to be highly motivated to learn. This motivation stems from a sense of personal achievement and the possibility of job advancement.

3. **Adults have competing demands for their time.** As adults, we have many different roles—spouses, parents, and workers, to name a few. These roles place demands on our time. You must be sensitive to these limitations. The failure of an EMT to attend a lecture off hours may not reflect a lack of commitment. Rather the EMT may be using that time to fulfill another role. Don't waste time. Be concise. Select required courses carefully. Don't expect a tremendous commitment of time away from work.

4. **Adults may lack confidence in their ability to learn.** Many adults have been away from the classroom for some time. Their study habits may be rusty, their reading ability diminished, and their attention span shortened. As a result your personnel may lack confidence in their ability to learn. To deal with this, make sure that your instructors give them frequent positive feedback.

5. **Adults within any group vary considerably.** If you instruct a group of fifth-graders, you will find that most are at about the same age, educational, and emotional level. The usual class of adult learners will vary more dramatically. When you plan courses, you will have dif-

ficulty using "one-size-fits-all" educational techniques. Direct your instructors to tailor their techniques to specific students.

These five factors characterize adult learners. Using them, you can develop a coherent approach to adult education. Unfortunately theory is not enough to guarantee success. You need to know how that theory applies to the real world of EMS education.

Education vs. training

A dramatic difference exists between education and training, and unless you understand that difference, you'll waste time and energy.[6] In general, education is directed at a broad base of knowledge that a person can apply to a variety of situations. Education is what physicians experience in their schooling. They receive a significant amount of general knowledge that isn't specifically applicable to a given set of circumstances. In EMS an educated person will assess an emergency, call on a body of knowledge, and develop an approach for dealing with the problem.

Training is different in that it identifies specific tasks that you want a person to perform. In EMS trained personnel will respond to an emergency by doing those things that they were trained to do. As such, training is more goal-oriented than education. In EMS there are far more trained people than educated people. EMTs, for example, are trained.

Establishing training programs

Because you'll direct most of your effort at training, you must learn how to establish training programs that meet your needs. Two steps are critical. First, you must determine what it is you want to do. When you developed your service's objectives in Chapter 2, you may have decided to upgrade prehospital care to the paramedic level. When you organized your service, you may have determined that you need six paramedics to achieve this. If your personnel are not at the paramedic level, you need to train them.

Second, evaluate your personnel to determine whether it will be possible to train them to the level that you've chosen. This involves determining where they are (in terms of training, attitude, and time responsibilities) and what their potential is (in terms of intelligence, training opportunities, and opportunities for skill maintenance). Continuing the paramedic example, if it's feasible that your personnel can move to the paramedic level, then training can go forward. If it is not feasible, then your objectives are probably unattainable with your current personnel.

Setting medical performance standards

Once you've completed these two steps, you need to integrate your training program with your EMS performance standards. That's one reason why it's important to have clear, written protocols. (We discuss protocols in detail in Chapter 9.) You must ask yourself: "What is it exactly that I want this person to do when the training is completed?" From there it's fairly simple to determine exactly what you must cover in your training program. You evaluate the current performance level of your personnel and subtract that from the performance level that you want to achieve. The result is what you must teach.

The training program

Once you've set your performance standards, you can begin to design the training program more specifically. Consider the appropriate training style, for example. Do you lecture? Do you encourage participation? As a general rule, EMS personnel tend to be tolerant of lectures. They appreciate demonstrations more. And if they can get their hands dirty, they learn the most. For this reason you should encourage hands-on experience whenever possible.

You train people to your performance objectives. The objectives should list exactly what you want your personnel to do when the training is over. Be sure that your students understand these objectives at the outset to ensure that they know what's expected of them. Then be certain that your examination process tests those objectives.

Selecting a trainer

Delegating the responsibility of the actual training to another person makes good sense. Conducting training programs is not a management function. For many EMS managers the time requirements of teaching become so extensive that the manager may have little time for more important functions. To be able to delegate the training role, however, you must select the right person.

In virtually every EMS organization there are likely to be people who, if given the opportunity, would be excellent trainers. Effective trainers must know the material that they are teaching and understand student motivation. Excellent models exist for developing EMS trainers.[7] In general, though, when you select trainers, think about the instructors who most influenced you; then find someone who possesses these same qualities. Effective instructors are usually dynamic, credible, and knowledgeable.

Summary

In order to achieve the goals and objectives that you developed for your service in Chapter 2, you must organize your personnel competently. To do that, you must understand how your service fits into the larger EMS system, determine how your service itself will be organized, and fit your service's jobs into that organization. In this chapter you learned the key principles and skills that you need for this kind of effective personnel organization.

Organizing your personnel is the first nuts-and-bolts step that you must take to make your service's goals and objectives reality. The second step is to make sure that you have the money to pay for the staff, equipment, and supplies that you need. That's the topic of Chapter 4.

4

Organizing your finances

EMS managers must understand that there is more to managing in EMS than just offering a service to the public responding to what happens. They must ensure that there are financial resources available to pay for the scope of services they envision. They must attempt to diversify their funding so they are not completely reliant on one source of income. EMS financial planning is difficult, but it is extremely important if systems are going to be successful.

—CHAIRMAN, FINANCE COMMITTEE OF REGIONAL EMS COUNCIL

Money is the necessary commodity that enables EMS goals to become reality. No matter how well you select your service's goals and organize your personnel, you won't accomplish much unless you have the money to fund what you're trying to do. As a result you *must* become an effective financial manager.

We can't teach you how to become a financial wizard in one chapter. In fact, if you are like many EMS managers, you may already be dreading this discussion. "Here it comes," you might be thinking. "I'm going to be buried in numbers and financial jargon." Most EMS managers entered EMS because they liked patient care. They were promoted because they were good at patient care. But once they become managers, they must deal with money. Often they do it reluctantly, saying "If I wanted to spend the day looking at numbers, I would have become an accountant."

In this chapter we'll teach you how to think about money and how to organize your finances. Don't worry if you don't know the difference between a debit and a credit. You still won't know the difference at the end of this chapter. We're not interested in jargon. We're interested in concepts. If you need to function as an accountant in your EMS management role, you may need to consider enrolling in a finance or accounting course to learn further details of the concepts that we're presenting here. But for most EMS managers the concepts provided here will enable them to organize their financial resources efficiently.

Learning from past mistakes

The federal Emergency Medical Services Systems grants played a major role in the development of EMS. Now the grant money is gone, forcing EMS managers to scramble for ever-decreasing sources of revenue. To learn to organize your service's financial resources effectively, you will find it helpful to examine two other federally funded health care programs to see the financial problems that they encountered. This will help you avoid those problems for your emergency medical service.[1]

Neighborhood health centers

In the late 1960s Lyndon Johnson's War on Poverty sought to improve health care delivery in poor neighborhoods by the development of neighborhood health centers (NHCs). The Office of Economic Opportunity (OEO) developed the NHCs, seeing them as one-stop providers of primary health care that would be easily accessible to the community. The OEO guidelines stipulated that a committee of community advisers and medical personnel aid in the development of the centers and ultimately assume their management.

The OEO provided the initial start-up money and expected that Medicaid and Medicare funds would be adequate to meet the centers' ongoing needs. Unfortunately Medicaid and Medicare funding proved inadequate. As a result, when OEO funding ended, the NHCs developed huge deficits. Many centers closed; others drastically reduced services.

The NHC concept did not die, however. It survives as the community health centers program funded by the Public Health Service. The fundamental difference between the two programs is that the Public Health Service provides direct ongoing support of approximately $400 million yearly. Thus the optimism of the 1960s that poor neighborhoods could sustain neighborhood health centers without continuing federal support has changed to the reality of the 1980s, where ongoing federal subsidies are essential to the program's survival.[2]

Will EMS systems go the route of the neighborhood health centers? One similarity between the two programs was the insistence by federal officials that the EMSS grants, like the OEO grants, were seed money—not intended for ongoing funding. To ensure that ongoing funding is adequate to meet system needs, the EMS manager must assess whether financial resources are available to meet the type and scope of services to be provided. As an EMS manager, you must live by the following rule:

New programs must make financial as well as medical sense.

Unfortunately many managers fail to plan adequately for the costs of new programs. In our region, for example, we never performed an evaluation of the ongoing costs of upgrading prehospital care under the EMSS grants. As a result we were unprepared for the 20 percent jump in prehospital salary costs that accompanied the transition to advanced life support. This led to a hasty, belated financial analysis of the whole system.

Lack of financial planning isn't the only factor threatening the long-term viability of EMS systems. The government's increasing fiscal conservatism is drying up anticipated funding sources. At the same time federal grants were ending, states began cutting back on funding as well; one state, for example, decided to limit its payment per ambulance run to approximately 40 percent of the cost of a routine advanced-life-support ambulance service call. This is typical of the nationwide trend in health care reimbursement on both the state and federal levels.

Health maintenance organizations

A second federally sponsored health program is worth examining. In 1973 Congress passed the Health Maintenance Organization (HMO) Act, which was to stimulate the development of HMOs. It offered start-up grants for new HMO programs and required employers of 25 or more that contributed to employee health plans to include a "federally qualified" HMO plan as an option if one were available. By 1979 only 51 of the 164 plans were "federally qualified." By 1980 several federally qualified plans were bankrupt and closed. The HMO Act of 1973 failed to stimulate much needed development because it placed unrealistic burdens on new plans, such as comprehensive around-the-clock treatment and open enrollment. The cost of meeting these regulations was more than some plans could bear.[3]

Has there been a similar development of unrealistic regulations in EMS? Perhaps there has. Clearly there are marked system-to-system differences. As funding becomes scarce, however, meeting certain regulations in EMS may become more difficult. In one state a group of small, volunteer ambulance services successfully lobbied for a bill in the legislature that limited the amount of training required for an entry-level ambulance attendant. Increasing educational requirements threatened the services' survival. This is an example of why you must constantly scrutinize regulations to see which are counterproductive.

Our point in evaluating these two programs isn't that federally sponsored programs always fail. In fact, both the neighborhood health centers and the HMO Act of 1973 have had notable successes. Rather the point is that past federally sponsored programs have suffered from government's overestimation of the local community's ability to develop financial support for health programs and its unrealistic imposition of regulations. As you look to the future, you must realize that these two problems are likely to threaten your service, and you must develop sound financial planning to overcome them.

Understanding costs

One concept that you must understand if you are to organize your finances competently is that of costs. To be able to think about costs effectively, you must understand the following topics:

1. Fixed costs vs. variable costs
2. Total costs vs. unit costs
3. Relevant costs vs. irrelevant costs
4. Opportunity costs
5. The time value of money

Fixed costs vs. variable costs

Fixed and variable costs differ in how they change in relation to a chosen activity or quantity. For example, suppose that you manage an ambulance service and wish to analyze your costs of medical supplies in relation to your daily number of runs. You would probably expect that the more runs per day, the greater the costs of medical supplies. As such, medical supplies are a variable cost with respect to number of runs. On the other hand, the heating bill for your station will be the same whether you see 10 or 100 patients in a day. Your heating costs are a fixed cost with respect to the number of runs.

Knowing what costs are fixed and what costs are variable helps you determine what your costs will be under certain circumstances. For example, if you're considering expanding your ambulance service's coverage area, variable costs like medical supplies will rise in response to the increased runs. Your fixed costs, like heating, will remain unchanged. This information can be helpful in determining whether expanding your service area makes financial sense.

Total costs vs. unit costs

When considering a decision where costs are an issue, you will generally want to consider total costs. Sometimes, however, you may need to consider unit costs. Suppose that you were considering the rental of a portable nitrous oxide unit for your ambulance. Although you feel that the device would improve the quality of patient care, you are concerned that because so few patients would use it, you wouldn't be able to recover the rental price through patient charges. (Let's assume that the unit rents for $500/year, and because of neighboring competition, you don't feel you can charge more than $5 per patient use.) If you restrict your analysis to examining total costs ($500), you will have difficulty making a decision. You must investigate unit costs in this instance, developing your best estimate for the number of patient uses that your service is likely to encounter. Suppose that you predict 25 patient uses for the coming year. A total cost of $500 divided by 25 uses yields a unit cost of $20. Clearly you will lose money on this rental if you can charge only $5 per use. On the other hand, if you estimate 250 uses per year, the unit cost would be $2, and the rental sounds much more appealing given the $5 charge per use.

In this example, knowing the total cost was not enough. You needed information on usage in order to calculate unit costs. These unit costs in turn enabled you to make the proper decision.

Relevant costs vs. irrelevant costs

Managers are decision makers. As a manger, you will find accounting information important in making the right decision among several alternatives. This does not mean, however, that all cost information is relevant to the decision at hand. Sometimes cost information is irrelevant and you should ignore it. A good example of this is the case of past (or "sunk") costs. Suppose that five years ago your service paid $6,000 for a new monitor. You currently pay $1,000 a year for a maintenance agreement on it, which covers all parts and labor. You learn of a new monitor of equal quality (given your service's needs), which, because of miniaturization of internal parts, costs only $2,000. The warranty on this new monitor covers parts and labor for one year, after which you could obtain a maintenance agreement for $200 a year. From a cost standpoint are you better off keeping the old monitor or purchasing the new one?

In this case the original purchase price of $6,000 five years ago is a past cost and is irrelevant to the decision. That money was spent and is irretrievable. As such you should not consider it in your decision. Rather you should decide based strictly on what each of these monitors will cost. Over the next five years you'll pay either $5,000 for service on the old monitor or $2,800 for purchase and service of the new monitor. From this perspective the new monitor is your best bet.

We are often resistant to this type of decision. After all, junking or selling the old monitor may seem a waste of $6,000. The point is that the $6,000 is gone forever, no matter what you decide.

Opportunity costs

Past costs, as we have just described, are real costs that should have no bearing on your future decisions. Opportunity costs represent the opposite concept. An opportunity cost is actually a nonexistent cost. Simply stated, an opportunity cost is the cost of *not doing* the next best alternative.

Suppose that your EMS responsibilities include managing an emergency department that operates a plaster room for applying casts. Your medical staff is interested in opening an endoscopy room, but the only way you can squeeze it into your current layout is to eliminate the plaster room and send fracture cases to the hospital across the street. Your medical staff estimates that you can earn an extra $200 a day from the endoscopic procedures. Should you pass up this revenue? The answer lies in the opportunity costs of eliminating the plaster room. If your plaster room brings in $175 a day, the true financial benefit of the endoscopy room is not really $200, but rather the endoscopy revenue minus the cost of the next best alternative, or $200 − $175 = $25.

Opportunity costs would be even more significant in this case if you were earning $250 a day from your plaster room. In this case the opportunity cost of the plaster room would be even greater than the income from the endoscopy room. From a financial perspective the decision to close the plaster room in such a case would be a poor one.

The time value of money

One of the more critical corollaries of the opportunity cost concept is the time value of money. This idea is important because you can generally invest money that you don't spend on new equipment or services. For that reason you must compare the return on your money from the new services with the return that you would receive if you invested it.

When you evaluate your service's finances, you must remember the time value of money. You'll quickly recognize several useful spinoffs of this concept. You should be wary, for example, of carrying excessively high levels of inventory, particularly for your more expensive supplies. An inventory item does not yield a financial return until it is sold. If your inventory level of synthetic casting material is so high that a $100 box of cast tape has sat on the shelf collecting dust for a year, you have incurred an opportunity cost of $12 if the interest rate at the bank were 12 percent. At the end of the year the material would still be worth $100 (assuming that there had been no price increase); on the other hand, if you had invested the $100 in the bank a year ago, it would be worth $112 today. Even more importantly you might have used the $100 to fund some other activity yielding an even higher return or a real benefit to patient care. Carrying excessive receivables works in much the same way. It is far better for a patient who owes you $100 to pay you today rather than a year from now. Money in your pocket today can be invested to yield a greater amount tomorrow.

Budgeting

When you develop a budget, you determine whether the goals that you developed in Chapter 2 and the personnel organization that you designed in Chapter 3 are financially feasible. In addition you determine how to organize your resources so that your money goes as far as possible. The best EMS managers wring every bit of performance from every dollar they have.

When you budget, you do three important things:

1. You force yourself to think concretely about the future and the financial implications of your service's goals. If, for example, your goal is to expand your ambulance coverage into a neighboring town, you must budget what you expect to earn and spend on this expansion. How much will you incur in additional salary or equipment costs? Budgeting forces you to consider key financial questions like this before you actually start spending money. For example, budgeting could alert you to the fact that under even ideal circumstances expanding your ambulance service's territory will result in a heavy financial loss. Obviously you must make such determinations *before* you act.

2. The budgeting process establishes the foundation for a system of financial analysis. The basic idea is this: As an EMS manager, you want to develop extremely accurate

predictions of future performance so that you can use those projections to answer such questions as: *Is my service doing as much business as expected? Am I paying for my personnel and materials what I expected to pay? Are my personnel as productive as I expected?* The budgeting process provides the first part of this analysis—the standard. In Chapter 10 we'll show you how you can compare actual performance to the standard to determine the answers to these questions through a process called *variance analysis.*

3. The budgeting process can improve communication within your service if you involve your employees. It can inform your personnel of your service's costs and generate enthusiasm for achieving standards.

You must complete four steps in order to forecast your service's finances:

1. Preparation for budget development
2. Projection of service volume
3. Development of expense forecast
4. Development of revenue forecast

Preparation for budget development

Before you can actually begin developing your budget, you must gather together several critical pieces of information. Specifically you need records of volumes of service, revenues, and costs for at least the last three years. If you don't have that information, start keeping it now. Historical data of this kind are crucial if you are going to develop an accurate budget. Your success as a financial manager depends on your ability to predict accurately future trends and the financial implications of your management decisions. If you don't have an accurate data base from which to predict future trends, your predictions will be inaccurate and you'll get into financial trouble fast.

Projection of service volume

In the last chapter we discussed a unit of work in EMS (for example, a patient visit or an ambulance run). When you develop your budget, you must have the ability to forecast accurately how many units of work your service will perform during the budget period.

Assuming that you have access to historical data, you should be able to make a reasonable prediction of future service. Say, for example, that you manage a private ambulance service and are trying to develop a volume projection for the upcoming year. If you plotted on a graph your service's number of runs for each of the last 15 years, the graph might look like Figure 4–1.

What you want to do with this graph is to draw the "best line" through the dots, which represents the underlying trend during the historical period. Extrapolating the line into next year gives you a forecast of service volume for that period. If you don't have access to a computer, you'll draw a straight line, leaving about an equal number of dots above and below the line. If you have a computer, you can use a technique called *linear regression*, which mathematically determines the best line and expresses it as a formula. [Excellent references are available on the regression technique.[4]]

There are two principles that you must follow in developing your forecast of future service.

1. **Be conservative.** One of the major causes for financial difficulties in EMS is wildly optimistic estimates of growth. If you overestimate growth, you're likely to hire more personnel and buy more equipment than you need. Once you realize that your estimates are high, it is

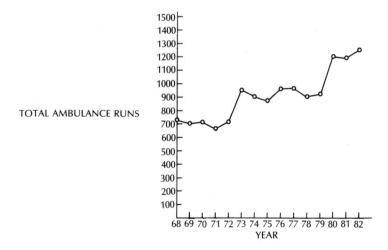

FIGURE 4-1. Total Ambulance Runs by Year

almost impossible to reduce your staffing and return your unnecessary equipment. It is much better to be conservative in your estimates. In that way, if you find that your actual volume of service exceeds your projection, you can increase your personnel and equipment; you don't spend money on those increases until you actually need to.

2. **Be alert for new trends.** A new ambulance service starting in a nearby town will almost certainly affect your volume of service. So will a new nursing home. You must be alert to these developments and adjust your forecasts accordingly. If you expect major changes in your service area and have access to a computer, you can design computer models to predict changes in volume.

Accurately forecasting volume is the most important step in the budget process. Because many of your costs and revenues vary as your volume of work changes, errors in your volume forecasts will result in inaccurate cost and revenue forecasts.

Development of expense forecast

Your expense forecast has three major parts: salaries, supplies, and equipment.

Salaries

Salaries generally represent at least half your costs. For this reason you must budget this expense accurately. This is relatively simple if you adopt a job-grading system.

To develop a job-grading system, first decide exactly which factors common to all jobs in your service should be included in the grading. Most organizations include factors such as education, experience, complexity of duties, responsibility for preventing errors, and work conditions. Let's suppose that you decide to use these five factors in a job-grading system.

After selecting the factors, you decide the importance of each factor. Perhaps you feel that in your organization experience is twice as important as education. You need to assign points to each factor to reflect this relative importance. You might assign a maximum of 20 points for experience and only 10 points for education. You then total the maximum number of points possible. The result might look like this:

Experience	20
Educational level	10
Complexity of duties	25
Errors	20
Working conditions	10
TOTAL	85

Next you must convert your point totals into labor grades. You'll want to establish a point range for each labor grade. In this example, if you were to have six labor grades, you might design them as follows:

Grade 1	5–15 points
Grade 2	16–30 points
Grade 3	31–44 points
Grade 4	45–60 points
Grade 5	61–72 points
Grade 6	73–85 points

You can then peg each job to a specific grade by the job's point total for the five factors. To do this, each factor is broken into a series of degrees. For example, degree 1 in education might be "basic knowledge of arithmetic, reading, and grammar...," while degree 3 might be "thorough knowledge of a specialized field, such as paramedicine or registered nursing...." Each degree has a point value attached to it. When you evaluate a job such as a paramedic, you would place it in degree 3 in the area of education. That degree might be worth 7 points. You then do the same thing for the other factors and add up the numbers that you assigned. For example, for a paramedic, you might end up with a score of 62, which would place the paramedic in grade 5.

Within each grade you also need to establish steps through which an employee advances based on predetermined factors (usually merit, tenure, or a combination of both). This advancement recognizes that the employee is developing increasing skill each year, thus delivering a greater level of performance.

As a final step you determine how much you are going to pay as an hourly rate for each step within each grade.

"Well, it didn't last very long," you might be saying. "You promised to stay away from jargon and now you're presenting a complex system of how to pay people. I run a small ambulance service, have two basic EMTs, and don't intend to either upgrade my service or expand. Why do I need a complicated grading system like this?" You don't. In some cases, like small ambulance services, grading systems are more trouble than they are worth. But for most EMS situations such systems are vital. Here's why:

1. **Grading systems ensure fairness.** If you have only one type of employee and each employee has about the same experience, you don't need a grading program because you'll pay everyone about the same. However, as soon as you have more than one type of employee or different experience levels, you must develop a system that ensures that you pay all your employees fairly.

2. **Grading enables you to predict the cost of changing the level of service that you offer.** One common mistake of EMS managers has been to underestimate the cost of upgrading a service's skill level. If you manage a service that does not operate at the highest training level possible, you have probably been asked to upgrade the service to a higher skill level. How do you determine the cost? If you have a job-grading system, you can grade the proposed higher skilled job and determine exactly how much you are going to pay. In this way you can accurately assess the financial impact of upgrading skills before you commit to doing it.

3. **Grading lets you correctly predict the financial impact of rewarding experience and merit.** Most EMS services pay more for experience or merit. If you manage in such a system, you need a reliable way of predicting how this practice will affect your budget. Through the job-grading system you accurately determine the impact of rewarding experience and merit by calculating how an employee's movement up a ladder of pay steps over the next year will affect your budget. You should carefully perform this calculation for each employee in your service.

Equipment and supplies

Budgeting for equipment is risky, because equipment purchases are generally expensive and made to satisfy needs over a long period. If you don't budget for the proper equipment, at the proper time, for the proper price, your service will have problems.

When you budget for equipment, you must gather as much objective information as possible. You need that information to answer the fundamental question: *What equipment is necessary to meet my service's goals and objectives?*

Table 4–1 contains a form to help you gather some of the information that you need to evaluate your equipment needs.

Your needs for equipment should follow the goals and objectives that you determined for your service in Chapter 2. Suppose that you manage an ambulance service and your top priority is to expand into a neighboring town at its request. Having established this objective, you may determine that you need a new ambulance.

When you evaluate equipment purchases, it's critical that you determine whether the proposed equipment meets a real

TABLE 4–1. Equipment Evaluation Form

Provide the following information for each piece of equipment requested:

1. A brief evaluation of the item, including the types of procedures to be done and where the item will be located in your service.

2. Whether the item is to be used for direct patient care.

    If so:

    a. Explain the improvement in health care provided by the machine.
    b. A charge per procedure.

    If not:

    a. Explain how the item will better satisfy the needs of the service.
    b. Whether any man-hours of labor will be saved by the item.

3. Whether the item is new or a replacement.

    If a replacement:

    a. Age of original equipment.
    b. Record of service repairs on the original item.
    c. New advances incorporated into replacement.
    d. The salvage value of equipment being replaced.

    In either case:

    a. Number of procedures that will use the item.
    b. Cost of the new item.
    c. Expected life of the new item.
    d. Whether any rearrangement will be necessary to accommodate the item.

need, not just an employee want. For example, some of your employees might want annual replacement of all your service's ambulances. It is unlikely that this replacement is necessary for you to achieve your service's objectives. Your real need is for dependable vehicles to transport patients in emergencies. Annual replacement of vehicles might be nice, but it can't be considered a real need.

It's impossible to consider every single supply need when you formulate your budget. You can develop a relatively accurate supply budget in the following way. Of all your service's costs, supplies are probably the most variable in nature; that is, there is usually a direct relationship between supplies and volume of service. For this reason you can use your volume projection in forecasting your supply costs. The actual calculation is easy:

$$\frac{\text{Current yr. supply cost}}{\text{Current yr. volume}} \times \frac{\text{Projected}}{\text{volume}} \times \text{Inflation} = \frac{\text{Forecasted}}{\text{supply cost}}$$

Your inflation factor should represent a best guess based on likely price increases and current economic conditions. You should consider other factors, such as technological changes or anticipated changes in services, that may affect the validity of your historical data. Estimate their impact on supplies and add them into your calculation.

Development of revenue forecast

Your total revenue forecast is directly dependent on your volume of service. Once you have made your volume forecast, your preliminary revenue forecast becomes easy:

$$\frac{\text{Current year revenue}}{\text{Current year volume}} \times \frac{\text{Projected}}{\text{volume}} = \frac{\text{Preliminary}}{\text{revenue forecast}}$$

This forecast is preliminary because it considers only changes in volume between the current year and the budget year. It doesn't consider changes in the rates that you charge for your services. Your service's rate changes will have a significant impact on your service's revenue. If your organization is to survive, you must set your rates so that you generate enough money to cover your costs. Although this sounds easy, it's often extremely tricky and explains why many EMS managers become prematurely gray.

Unlike most businesses, what you charge in EMS is unlikely to equal what you collect. Many patients carry insurance, which covers part, if not all, of their health care needs. This insurance may be government-sponsored, such as Medicare or Medicaid, or private, such as Blue Cross. In addition, many EMS services are provided by or for city or county governments. Each of these groups is likely to pay for your services according to its own rules; many link their payments to your costs.

The more informed you are about these rules (and they change all the time) and about your general mix of patients according to payor, the more accurate you'll be in predicting how certain changes in your rate structure will influence your total revenue. If, for example, you find that Medicare, Medicaid, and Blue Cross in your state reimburse you roughly the equivalent of costs that you incur in treating their patients (regardless of your rate) and that together they cover 75 percent of your patients, then a one dollar increase in charge per patient will generate only 25 cents more revenue. Clearly you must include this type of information in your total revenue forecast if it is to be accurate.

A second factor that you must consider when you increase your rates is the public reaction. This is particularly important if you compete with several alternative services in your local area. Unless you can convey to the public that your service is superior in quality to your competitors', you can't charge more without risking a loss of business.

Even if your service enjoys a relative monopoly in your community, you must be careful when you increase your rates. The general public is aware of rising health care costs, particularly during periods when it is a "hot" political issue. If you manage an ambulance service and have established an advisory committee of private citizens, as suggested in Chapter 2, you will want to review your proposed rate changes with them to assess the public's reaction. If the public views your rate increases as unwarranted, you may cause a backlash of adverse publicity, which will decrease your volume of service. This might more than offset the increased revenue that the higher rates will generate.

From this discussion you can see that rate setting for your service can be a difficult issue. Each specific EMS service operates under its own set of circumstances. As an EMS manager, you must accurately assess how reimbursement rules, local competition, and public opinion will affect your rate structure. Only then can you make a final revenue forecast.

When you have completed these four steps (preparation, volume projection, expense projection, and revenue projection), you can determine whether the revenues that you intend to generate will cover your expenses. If you find that your revenues fall short, you'll have to reevaluate your service's objectives and scale them back.

Two final items that you need to know

As we've presented it, the budgeting process works well. But it works even better if you add two tools.

Zero-base budgeting

You can simplify the process of establishing your salary, supply, and equipment expense forecasts if you merely use last year's actual costs plus an inflation factor and information about projected changes in your service. Many EMS managers do that, limiting their justifications for the final forecasts to the incremental portion alone (the portion that exceeds last year's actual costs). In this way they need only defend the increase over the previous year's appropriations. They accept what they are already spending without question. Thus any inefficiencies reflected in prior costs will appear in future forecasts.

You'll manage more effectively if you use zero-base budgeting, where you start from scratch every year in developing expense forecasts. Although this requires more work, you may uncover unjustified costs and inefficiencies from the past that you might overlook without the zero-base approach.

Responsibility accounting

When developing budgets, how much detail is necessary? You can adopt a simple approach, generating one budget for your entire service. If you have a small service, this might be adequate. However, if you rely on this method in a larger service, you'll miss an important aspect of budgeting: responsibility accounting.

If you manage a larger service, various centers are probably responsible for specific expenditures. Perhaps you manage an emergency department and three ambulance services. You em-

ploy a separate supervisor for each of these major divisions.
Each supervisor makes decisions regarding cost issues in his
area. In a case like this you can improve the budgeting process if
you work with your supervisors to develop individual budgets
for each of these areas. You can then provide each supervisor
with regular feedback on performance by comparing budget to
actual performance. In this way you trace costs to the individual
who has primary responsibility for them. If you manage a service
with several cost areas, develop a budget network that mirrors
the actual decision-making structure. This generally costs little
and will markedly improve the entire budgeting process.

Purchasing

Earlier in this chapter we discussed budgeting for equipment
and supplies. Although effective budgeting in these areas is necessary to ensure the proper financial management of your service, it alone isn't sufficient. You must also ensure that you actually spend your service's dollars wisely in acquiring equipment
and supplies during the year. This is not always easy. What do
you do, for example, when one of your staff shows you an ad for a
defibrillator and requests that you order one? If that defibrillator is necessary to meet your service's goals and objectives,
then consider evaluating this request further. If its purchase
would meet only an employee's want, don't pursue it.

It's unlikely that available funds can match the total of all
the legitimate needs of your service. As a result you must weigh
the relative merits of your needs and satisfy only the most important. In general you should first attempt to satisfy those needs
that are most consistent with your service's highest priority
goals.

When you've determined that a request meets a high priority
need, you should evaluate the item itself to make sure that it lives
up to its promise. You can briefly evaluate a new item right at
your desk, screening out products that fall short of your standards. Perhaps a new defibrillator is so bulky that it would take a
weight lifter to carry it around all day. The evaluation need go no
further. If, however, your examination of the product reveals no
obvious defects, you should then test the item in the field, where
it will undergo the actual conditions for which it was intended.
Inform your staff of the nature of the evaluation and determine

with them a suitable time frame for the test. At the conclusion of the evaluation period, seek feedback from your staff concerning all aspects of the product. Table 4–2 provides a useful product evaluation form for this. Using this form ensures that you ask the right questions.

After you've determined that a supply item or piece of equipment truly meets one of your service's needs, you should evaluate

TABLE 4–2. Product Evaluation Form

TO: _____ PRODUCT: _____

FROM: _____ COMPANY: _____

PLEASE RETURN EVALUATION BY: _____

THIS PRODUCT IF ACCEPTABLE WILL REPLACE: _____

NOTE: Please use this product and be objective in your evaluation.

I. Were the samples of this product:

  Accompanied by proper instructions?   YES   NO

  Sufficient in number for an adequate evaluation?   YES   NO

II. Is this product easier to use than the one we are currently using?   Harder to use?   Similar?   Give reasons:

_____

_____

III. Is this product more effective than the one we are currently using?   Less effective?   Similar?   Give reasons:

_____

_____

IV. Does this product improve patient care?   YES   NO

  Does it make your job easier?   YES   NO

  Comments: _____

_____

V. Do you recommend we should change to this product?   YES   NO

VI. Do you foresee any problem with changing?   YES   NO

  If yes, please explain: _____

_____

reliability, service, and availability. The best piece of equipment may become a worthless piece of junk if you can't obtain competent service. All these steps must be taken before you determine whether you are getting the best price, because *a bad purchase, at any price, is a bad purchase.* No matter how inviting the price may be, if the quality is lacking or the product is not available when you need it, you can't afford it. It simply won't satisfy your needs.

In Chapter 6 we will describe techniques to improve your bargaining position in a negotiation. You can purchase equipment and supplies at better prices if you routinely apply two of those techniques: creating competition and forming coalitions.

You can ensure that you receive the best price if you encourage competitive bidding between vendors. Once you've determined the lowest bid, you should develop a written agreement with the vendor for the needed item, fixing the price for a set period. Although this limits your flexibility to make changes in products, you can avoid many time-consuming elements of purchasing (such as evaluations) for long periods. You can coordinate the evaluations of competing products by scheduling them at a point three or four months before your existing agreement ends. Not only does this streamline the evaluation process, but it promotes head-to-head competition between products to highlight the relative merits of each. This competitive process generally lowers prices.

A second means of lowering prices is group purchasing, where individual organizations band together to gain greater bargaining strength by pooling their purchases. Although the first hospital purchasing group began early in the twentieth century, the concept has just recently begun to catch fire. Virtually every state has a group of health care institutions that collectively establishes contracts on everything from underpads to IVs. Although these groups are composed primarily of hospitals and are often organized as an arm of a state or regional hospital association, many extend membership to affiliated health care providers such as independent ambulance services and nursing homes in order to increase the purchasing base, and thus the bargaining strength, of the full group.

Entry fees into group purchasing organizations are generally quite low. Most organizations assess the fee annually, based on size of service. As a result the entry fee for a small ambulance service is minimal, particularly in comparison to the potential savings in purchased supplies.

Given the low costs and potential benefits of group purchasing, you should investigate the possibility of your service's joining such a group. A call to your state hospital association should provide you with information concerning the nature of groups in your area.

Summary

The proper management of your service's financial resources is more critical today than ever before. Applying principles of financial organization outlined in this chapter should assist you in this effort. You can achieve nothing as a manager unless you have the money to pay for it. However, if you combine effective planning and personnel organization with sound finances, you are ready to pursue your service's goals successfully. To translate plans and organization into action, you need to be able to direct your service through the obstacles that stand between you and successful performance. In the last two chapters you learned the nuts and bolts of organization. In the next section you'll learn the key principles of directing.

III

DIRECTING

This section presents the essentials of effective direction.

Chapter 5, "Improving Your Ability to Communicate," reviews the barriers to communication and suggests methods to overcome them. It also introduces you to active listening techniques and verbal assertiveness skills.

Chapter 6, "Negotiating," covers the principles of competent negotiating. Successes and failures of actual EMS negotiations are reviewed in order to illustrate sound negotiating principles.

Chapter 7, "Learning to Delegate," discusses the nature of delegation, ways to use it effectively, and reasons why EMS managers often fail to delegate well. Delegation is a time-management skill essential to effective EMS management.

Chapter 8, "Directing Change," shows you why EMS managers are often unsuccessful when they try to introduce new programs. It reviews the nature of tasks, resistance, and power and shows you how to predict resistance to change and counteract it.

5

Improving your ability to communicate

Communication is the biggest problem in EMS. People just don't listen. Basically, they come to a meeting with their own perceptions of what's going on, they speak what's on their mind, and they leave with their own perceptions. There's no interchange of ideas.
—EMERGENCY DEPARTMENT DIRECTOR

In the first four chapters you've learned to plan and organize. Now you must improve your directing skills so that you can actually produce results through your personnel. The first step in improving your directing skills is for you to become a better communicator. If you've been around EMS management very long, you'll probably agree that poor communication is the reason most frequently cited for problems between people in EMS. "We must communicate better" seems to be the catch phrase of our age.

As a manager faced with communication problems, you'll probably try to solve them by having more meetings. Sometimes that works. Communication problems can occur because you are not communicating enough. Often, however, increasing the quantity of communication is not the answer; rather, you must improve the *quality* of communication. Better communication requires effective listening and assertive expression. In this chapter you'll learn the skills necessary to make all your communications better.

Improving your listening skills

We know what you're thinking. "A whole section on listening. What a drag!" You can probably think of a thousand more exciting topics for a section in a book. So can we. But the purpose of this book is to make you a better manager. You can either read this section now and save your personnel and yourself a lot of grief, or you can wait until you've made so many stupid moves that everyone around you becomes convinced that you're a hopeless case. If you don't listen well, you're headed for trouble. Our job is to help you avoid that trouble. To do that, you must improve your listening skills.[1]

How often have you heard this type of ineffective dialogue:

Chairman: The first item on today's agenda is the development of a capital budget.

Speaker 1:   We need more monitoring equipment. How are we supposed to handle a big emergency if we don't get equipment?

Speaker 2: We should set the long-range EMS goals first, then decide what equipment we need in the capital budget. That's the organized way to proceed.

Speaker 3: A television set for the emergency department waiting room would be good. The patients would really like that.

Speaker 4: We're just wasting our time! The administration is so tight, we'll never get what we ask for.

This sounds familiar, doesn't it? The problem here is that one speaker's opening words have little relation to the previous speaker's closing words. Even though all speakers have their own thoughts well-organized, there is little continuity of thought between speakers. The discussion hops from one idea to another without any direction. You've been in discussions like this, and if you're like most people, you quickly become frustrated. Everyone is "blowing off steam," but the group is going nowhere. No wonder meetings are often a waste of time.

Why does this problem exist? To a large extent poor communication results from poor listening skills. All too often *we hear the words but miss the message.*

Why don't we listen effectively? Some people decide not to listen because they consider listening to be a passive exercise and a sign of weakness. Indeed today's image of the macho EMS manager is someone who can give orders and crack a few heads together. In this view the manager is someone who is listened to, not someone who listens. EMS managers who adopt this style almost inevitably run into problems.

Many EMS managers want to listen but encounter problems along the way. One reason we have problems is that we have more time to listen than we really need. We can usually understand a speaker talking at a rate of 500 words per minute. The typical speaker, however, talks at a rate of about 250 words per minute. When we are listening, we need only half of the available time to comprehend the words (comprehension time). The other half (reaction time) exists for us to use as we like. The key to effective listening is to use this reaction time to your advantage. Poor listeners waste their reaction time or worse yet misuse it so that they fail to understand what they are hearing.

We're going to examine three types of listeners: the daydreamer, the dissonance reducer, and the active listener. The first type of listener uses reaction time for daydreaming; the second molds the message to his or her own attitudes, often distorting the speaker's message in the process; the third takes advantage of reaction time and thereby creates efficient and effective communication, which in turn produces workable solutions to problems.

The daydreamer

Daydreaming is not inherently bad; in fact it lets us use our imagination. However, if we lose control over when and how much we daydream, we risk missing important messages.

What factors cause us to begin daydreaming? Sometimes a message seems too simple to warrant the time that we would spend in listening. We become bored ("What else is new?") and use this to justify tuning the speaker out, even though the speaker may move into new subjects of potential interest. We daydream when a message seems too complex to understand. In these cases we become discouraged because we are beneath a speaker's intellectual level ("I'm completely lost!"). Rather than asking the speaker to simplify the message, we begin to daydream. This is particularly true when we are part of a large group. We don't want to ask a "stupid question" even though other audience members may be equally confused by the speaker's message.

Sometimes a speaker will use an emotionally charged word or phrase that makes us think of something completely irrelevant. Perhaps you cringe at the phrase *ambulance breakdown,* and when you hear it, you daydream about replacing all your vehicles with new models. By the time you realize you're daydreaming, you've lost the speaker's intended message.

Sometimes we're not exactly daydreaming but simply concentrating on something else, so that when a speaker approaches us, we don't even begin to listen. In this instance communication doesn't stand a chance.

The end result of these four communication problems is that we do not listen to the message. To solve them, we must concentrate on understanding what the speaker is trying to say. Listening is not a passive exercise; it requires work.

Note taking can assist you in maintaining your attention on what you are hearing. It can make you a better listener by forcing you to concentrate on the message closely enough to be able to express the speaker's key ideas in your own words. Notes can also be helpful if you don't trust your memory to remember what you are hearing. Make sure that your notes express your understanding of the message and your thoughts about it. Avoid merely copying down what the speaker is saying without thinking.

The dissonance reducer

A second type of listener is the dissonance reducer. Dissonance reduction is a more subtle communication problem than daydreaming.[2] Here's how it works: We all have certain attitudes and beliefs that we've developed through our life experiences. Often we are faced with information that contradicts our established attitudes. When we encounter this new information, we experience an internal conflict called *dissonance.* Because our minds usually dislike dissonance, we attempt to minimize it in a variety of ways. We can change our attitudes to make them more consistent with the new information, or we can deal with the new information in other ways, sometimes called *defense mechanisms.*

Rationalization, which is one type of defense mechanism, allows us to dispose of a message if we can "logically" (though incorrectly) convince ourselves that the message is wrong. Suppose, for example, that one of your duties is to purchase supplies, and you have been buying 5cc syringes from the Acme Company for 25 cents each. An EMT approaches you with an essentially identical syringe made by the Ajax Company and tells you that these can be purchased for 10 cents each. You're supposed to be getting the best deal possible, and now an EMT is showing you that you aren't—some nerve. You can accept what the EMT says and admit that you've been making a mistake. Alternatively you can continue to believe that you are getting the best deal possible on syringes if you can convince yourself that the 10-cent syringe is not identical to the 25-cent syringe and will not satisfy your needs. So you tell the EMT that the label on the cheaper syringe says 5cc in smaller print, and you're concerned that it will be difficult for everyone to read. So you won't switch. In this situation you used your reaction time counterproductively. Rather than using it to enhance the real message (namely, that some savings could be achieved), you used it to reduce the dissonance that you experienced when you realized that you were wrong.

A second way in which we use reaction time to reduce dissonance is to alter the incoming message. A filter in our brain screens messages for potential dissonance. This filter generally allows messages that are consistent with our established beliefs to pass through undistorted. Messages that generate dissonance, on the other hand, are changed so as to increase consistency with our established beliefs. Suppose, for example, that you are responsible for repairing portable radios and that two portable radios have been broken for some time. You have called the manufacturer repeatedly, but the necessary parts are temporarily out of stock. There is little that you can do about the situation, but you feel bad anyway. You pass a coworker in the hallway and he says, "Hey, have you got those radios fixed yet?" You mutter no and walk along fuming, "Why does he always pick on me?" If you asked the coworker why he questioned you, he might say that he'd passed you twice already in the hall that day and said hello. The third time he wanted to say something more personal, and because he knew that you were working on the radio problem, he asked you about it. Because you felt guilty already, you distorted the speaker's message so that it sounded like a criticism.

A third way in which we use reaction time to reduce dissonance is to deny (totally ignore) a message. Most of us practice denial with the messages of certain speakers. Perhaps you have a disgruntled employee who disregards everything that you say. Whenever you approach him, he responds with an automatic "Yeah, yeah, sure, Boss," while actually thinking "Is this creep trying to tell me how to do my job again?" You may practice denial if you have a "problem" employee. While the employee is unloading a gripe, you cease listening and start thinking, "Bitch, bitch, bitch! That's all I ever hear." Denial is an extremely effective way to reduce dissonance. If you strongly believe that the speaker has nothing of value to offer, you will never be challenged if you refuse to acknowledge any of the speaker's messages.

The subtlety of dissonance reduction makes it more difficult to manage than daydreaming. This is particularly true when the speaker's message deals with you personally. We are all accustomed to viewing ourselves in certain ways, subconsciously filtering to see and hear only what we want to see and hear. If you wish to overcome this, you must develop the ability to listen to yourself. You need to identify when your mind erects a defensive barrier in response to what someone is saying about you. When someone touches off feelings within you that block your attempts to listen, try to step back and listen to yourself. Try to understand those feelings so they don't prevent you from listening.

The active listener

Thus far we have identified two key elements in effective listening: paying more attention to the message and learning to listen to ourselves. We must go further, however. We need to sharpen our listening skills in order to achieve a higher capability called *active listening*.[3,4] Active listening requires that we listen with a greater degree of sensitivity. We can better understand what is being said if we sense how the speaker's statement actually feels to him. As a first step we must learn the distinction between a message's content and feeling.

Content refers to the meanings of the words themselves. We must be clear of the meanings within a message if we are to understand it fully. Although this may sound simple, sometimes we find ourselves confronted with unfamiliar terminology. Computer people are notorious in this regard; they often use computer jargon that is incomprehensible to 99 percent of us. Even with simple everyday phrases, we may find that a single word can have a variety of meanings. Think of a question like *did you see that check?* Depending on the context, *check* could take on one of more than 10 definitions. The speaker could be referring to a document from his bank, the design on a shirt, a maneuver in a hockey game, or a person from Czechoslovakia. To understand content, the listener may have to seek clarification to determine which definition the speaker has chosen.

Slightly different forms of the same statement can have virtually the same content. For example, the content of the statement *I'm leaving now*, is virtually the same as the content of the statement *I'm leaving this damned place right now*. Obviously, though, the two statements deliver different messages. This results from the different *feeling* of each.

To understand a speaker's feelings, you must pay attention to both nonverbal and verbal cues, because the speaker expresses feeling not only through words and tone of voice but also through facial expressions, eye movements, and body motions. During a conversation people normally look at each other 40 to 60 percent of the time. The nonverbal cues during that time convey a surprising amount of information. The interpretation of nonverbal cues or body language is an inexact science. Catalogues purport to describe the meaning of numerous gestures. Certain interpretations of body language seem reasonable. Table 5–1 lists 10 common interpretations of body language.

TABLE 5–1. Ten Key Body Language Cues

SPEAKER	MEANING
Avoids eye contact.	Dislike or disinterest.
Crosses arms across chest, tightly crosses legs, or straddles chair so that its back is between you.	A defensive signal. The speaker is nervous, uneasy, or holding out.
Leans back in chair, steeples fingers, and peers over them.	Sign of superiority. Speaker feels more powerful or knowledgeable than you.
Talks with hands open, palms facing upward.	Sign of sincerity. Speaker probably feels there is nothing to hide.
Tilts head.	Usually a sign that the speaker is listening intently to what you have to say.
Crosses legs. Moves foot back and forth in a kicking motion.	Bored or impatient. Probably isn't listening to you.
Suddenly shifts feet so they are headed toward the door. Maintains this position.	Ready to terminate conversation.
Drums fingers on desk top or taps feet on floor.	Bored or impatient. Better speed up what you are saying.
Leans forward, sits on edge of chair.	Interested. Ready for meaningful discussion or decision.
Smooths hair or pats it gently.	Sign of approval.

If you look for the body language cues listed in Table 5–1, you should be able to understand better the speaker's intent; because nonverbal cues are often subconscious, they are less likely to be disguised by the speaker. Consequently nonverbal cues may reveal true feelings.

Once we think that we understand both a message's content and feeling, we can test our understanding by using several active listening techniques.[5] These techniques, summarized in Table 5–2, direct us to explore the message further, ensuring our fuller understanding of it.

One technique, called *paraphrasing*, consists of rephrasing in your own words what you think the speaker means. This can be effective in testing and ensuring your understanding of a message's content. It also lets the speaker know that you are actively listening. For example, after listening to an EMT's com-

TABLE 5–2.   Active Listening Techniques

PARAPHRASING

Definition: Rephrase the speaker's message in your own words.

Purpose: Ensures you understand the message.

Example: "In other words, what you are saying is. . . ."

REFLECTION

Definition: Express your interpretation of a message's feeling rather than content.

Purpose: Tells the speaker you have recognized the feeling of the message; defuses negative feelings.

Example: "You sound really upset about this."

NEUTRAL

Definition: Use encouraging signals to keep the speaker talking.

Purpose: Encourages the speaker to provide a broader or more detailed message.

Example: "I see."

CLARIFICATION

Definition: Make a statement or question aimed at a specific point.

Purpose: Elicits a response to satisfy an unclear area.

Example: "Why do you say that?"

SUMMARIZATION

Definition: Link together several previous statements into one central idea.

Purpose: Helps organize a speaker's thoughts or a group dialogue.

Example: "Let's review what's been said up to now."

plaint about paper work, you might say, "So what you're saying is that if we could streamline our run report form, we'd save time and effort." By paraphrasing a speaker's message you will elicit a response from the speaker that should tell you whether the person feels properly understood. For example, the EMT might say,

"Yeh, that's right" or "Not only the run report form, but the vehicle check list as well."

A second technique, called *reflection*, is slightly different from paraphrasing. When you reflect on a speaker's message, you interpret the speaker's *feelings*, rather than paraphrasing the message's content. This is particularly useful as an initial response to a speaker who expresses strong feelings. Suppose, for example, that you are the head nurse in an emergency department, and an emergency department physician approaches you screaming, "These ER nurses are totally incompetent!" You might reflectively reply, "Sounds like you're mad as hell about something." Such a reply acknowledges the speaker's primary message—his feelings—and in so doing can diffuse the speaker's anger so that productive communication proceeds. Remember that a speaker may have difficulty in clearly expressing the "facts" of a message until feelings are acknowledged. Your recognition of these feelings by the reflective technique may provide just what the speaker needs. Remember, too, that in these cases nonverbal cues can provide useful information.

The *neutral* technique encourages a speaker to continue talking. A simple "Uh-huh" or a nod of the head is usually an effective signal that we are interested and are listening. Such responses prompt the speaker to continue.

The *clarifying* technique is used when we need further information of a specific nature. It usually consists of a question based on the speaker's previous statement. For example, if an EMT says, "That cardiac refresher course was terrible," you might say, "Was the whole course terrible or just some of the parts?" in order to clarify what course changes are appropriate.

A fifth technique, *summarization*, involves combining a speaker's thoughts into a concise statement that focuses on the speaker's key points. This technique can be particularly useful when applied to a group discussion, where statements of different individuals need to be combined. The dialogue concerning the EMS budget at the beginning of this section could be markedly improved by an active listener's summarization of the discussion. The listener might say: "It sounds like we have a real divergence of opinion here. Mary feels that we need new monitoring equipment. John wants a T.V. for the waiting room. Al questions whether we should bother spending our time developing a budget. Maybe we should first consider Sue's advice about further planning. Before we become embroiled in the specifics, we could examine both the history of the EMS capital budget and where it should go in the future. OK?" This approach ties the dialogue together and keeps all group members on the same track.

Assuming that you are successful, what are the benefits of active listening? As a speaker, you will speak more freely when you feel that listeners are trying to understand your message fully. Active listeners will encourage you to listen to yourself more closely and express yourself more clearly. As a listener, active listening can make you better informed. You ensure that you receive messages accurately and you can encourage the speaker to provide additional necessary information. From a group's point of view, active listening can lead to positive relationships, constructive attitude changes, and a greater probability of reaching workable solutions to problems. Misinterpretation of messages will diminish, and meetings will become more efficient. By listening to each other group members convey the idea that they are sincerely interested in each other and that they respect each other's thoughts (though not necessarily agreeing with them). In the final analysis the greatest benefit of active listening may be the simple fact that it tells speakers that they are worth listening to. This all-important element of recognition helps develop a relationship of trust, which in turn serves as a foundation for active mutual participation toward a greater common goal.

Learning to express your feelings effectively

Refining your listening ability is only half the battle in improving your communications. You must also learn to express effectively your own feelings and point of view. In short, you must assert yourself.

What is assertiveness? Strictly defined, "to assert oneself" means "to defend or maintain one's rights."[6] Why are we interested in assertiveness? Assertiveness is an effective method of handling certain aspects of your life. Assertiveness enables you to express your feelings, defend your opinions, and protect your rights without feeling defensive or guilty.

Assertiveness training encourages you to express your beliefs and feelings. It aids you in influencing the way that others behave toward you and assists others in better understanding your feelings. As such, assertiveness training is a positive step toward better communication for everyone concerned.

Assertiveness training has become popular recently. Why? Are we growing steadily less assertive over time? It's unlikely that we're any less assertive today than people 100 years ago. What has changed is our environment. The pace of life quickens a little more every year. Technology advances. Our expectations are increasing while our resources are diminishing. We experience greater stress and feel helpless because we aren't in complete control of where we are going. In order to cope, we must recognize our rights and feelings and learn how to stand up for them, for our environment becomes less forgiving each day to those of us who lack assertiveness.

To be an effective manager, you must be assertive. What would happen if you felt uneasy and guilty every time that you had to say no to an employee? How effective a representative of your service would you be if you couldn't stand up for your point of view in a regional meeting? What would be the impact on your home life if you couldn't assert your personal needs and allowed work demands to erode your time with your children? For these reasons and many others you must be assertive.

Few of us are naturally assertive. When it comes to defending one's rights, many people fall into one of two extremist categories of self-expression: aggressiveness or passivity. We are all born aggressive. As infants, we have no concept of the rights and needs of others. You can prove this point to yourself by watching a group of 18-month-old children play. Some people never develop beyond this point. These individuals hurt others, either emotionally or physically, as they engage in "I win/you lose" behavior. For others, certain life experiences (particularly parental relations) tend to mask this aggressiveness through the development of powerful inhibitions. Parental use of guilt and anxiety are effective measures of curbing aggressive behavior. Environments characterized by these emotions, however, often breed passive individuals whose inhibitions are so strong that they rarely express their own rights.

It is the rare individual whose life experiences have blended just the right mature ingredients to produce natural assertiveness: the ability to express one's own rights without denying that same freedom of expression to others. If you are such an individual, you don't need this section. If you're not, don't lose hope. You can learn assertiveness. The first step is to determine what your natural tendencies are so that you'll know where to direct your efforts at becoming more assertive. To determine your degree of aggressiveness, answer the following questions:

1. Do you control conversations?
2. Do you always think that you have the right answer?
3. Do you often step in and make decisions for others?
4. Do you continue to pursue an argument after the other person has had enough?
5. Are you prone to fly off the handle?
6. Do you show your anger by name calling and obscenities?
7. Do you shout or use bullying tactics to force others to do as you wish?
8. Do you physically fight with others?

Did you answer yes to any of these questions? If so, you probably exhibit a certain degree of aggressiveness. All of us have experienced aggressive managers—managers who are always "right," who step in and make all the decisions, and who threaten or bully us if we don't do as we're told. Aggressive managers are rarely effective managers.

The opposite of aggressiveness is passivity. Passivity can also limit your managerial effectiveness. To determine your degree of passivity, answer these questions:

1. When your meal is improperly prepared or served in a restaurant, do you ask the waiter to correct the situation?
2. When a salesman gives you a hard sell, do you say no if the merchandise is not what you want?
3. When you discover merchandise is faulty, do you return it for an adjustment?
4. If you are disturbed by someone smoking near you, do you say so?
5. When a latecomer is waited on before you, do you call attention to the situation?
6. If a person has borrowed money or a personal possession and is overdue in returning it, do you mention it?

7. When you disagree with a person whom you respect, do you speak up for your own viewpoint?

8. Do you refuse unreasonable requests made by friends?

Did you answer no to any of these questions? If so, you probably possess a certain amount of passivity, which may be a liability in situations where you need to stand up for your rights or your service's rights.

As a further test, let's examine three ways of dealing with a situation. Suppose that you are the director of a municipal ambulance service. Your boss is the supervisor of the Department of Public Safety. He is arrogant, opinionated, and powerful. No one likes to deal with him. You need to buy a new ambulance because yours is more rust than metal. Which of the following examples best describes how you would handle the situation?

Scene 1

You: Pardon me. Could I disturb you for a minute? Could we discuss the possibility of buying a new ambulance?

Supervisor: (thumbing through a magazine): Hey, how about another time?

You: Oh, sorry.

Scene 2

You: I'm getting tired of all your ambulances falling apart. We need a new one.

Supervisor: (thumbing through a magazine): Hey, how about another time?

You: I want to talk about it now. I'm getting tired of you putting me off. You don't give a damn whether things fall apart or not.

Supervisor: What are you talking about? I care! I just don't want to talk about it now. I....

You: Yeah, right. You guys in the office don't know what it's like on the street.

Supervisor: I was on the street before you were born. Get out of here, before I kick you out!

Scene 3

You:	Excuse me. I need to talk to you about buying a new ambulance.
Supervisor:	(thumbing through a magazine): Hey, how about another time?
You:	I think that this is a problem that we can't put off. I'm really getting worried about it.
Supervisor:	Sure, but do we have to discuss it now?
You:	I've already figured out a couple of ways we could go. I thought we could go over them. Maybe on Friday, over breakfast?
Supervisor:	Friday! I'm all jammed up on Friday. Do we have to. . . .
You:	Would you like another time?
Supervisor:	No. I guess not.
You:	Good, let's do it then. O.K.?
Supervisor:	Sure.
You:	Great. We'll both look pretty bad if something happens. This way we can prevent some problems. See you on Friday.

The three scenes are strikingly different. In the first scene the passive person opens with a request for a dialogue. The reply essentially ignores the request. The passive person doesn't pursue the issue further.

Nobody wins in an aggressive scene like the second one. Nothing is accomplished, either, and everyone feels bad about the way things turn out. Aggressive encounters usually result in a win-lose situation and weaken the relationship between the parties.

Assertive behavior doesn't establish win-lose situations but rather stresses negotiation of workable compromises. In the third scene, you have demonstrated many useful assertive skills. For one thing, you open with a clear statement of what you're interested in and why. You prepare potential options ahead of time and limit your request to a decision between those established options. That's helpful because you're more likely to succeed when your request is small rather than large. Establishing a mutually agreed time to discuss the matter assures that it will be addressed without pressuring the other person to cut short whatever he is doing now. And rewarding the other person with positive feedback is a healthy reinforcer.

The most striking difference between the assertive scene and the other two scenes is that it succeeded in solving the problem for which it was intended. This is the ultimate goal of assertive behavior.

Can techniques such as those described in the third scene be organized into a systematic framework of assertiveness? Yes, they can. Let's review some of the basics.

The first step in establishing a framework for assertiveness is to decide when to use the skills. Remember the 80/20 rule from Chapter 1; not all activities that you pursue are likely to be significant. Therefore, don't try to be assertive about everything. Many ideas aren't worth pursuing; many things that you don't like aren't worth the time it would take you to correct them. Besides, people stop listening if you talk all the time. We usually devote our greatest attention to those people who choose only the most important occasions to address an issue. Generally it pays to be an active listener all the time, but an effective speaker will pick and choose among opportunities.

Equally important, of course, is avoiding the opposite extreme: talking yourself out of being assertive in *every* situation because "it just isn't that important." Avoid both extremes by asking yourself the following questions:

1. How important is this issue to me?
   a. How will I feel if I do this?
   b. How will I feel if I don't do this?
2. How likely am I to succeed?
3. What are the benefits of success?
4. What are the costs of success?

Your answers to these questions should enable you to select those issues that warrant your time.

After you have identified when to be assertive, you need to learn how to be assertive. Two Stanford University psychologists have devised an approach to assertiveness that they call a DESC script.[7] DESC stands for describe, express, specify, and consequences. It is an outline for an organized, specific, assertive statement of facts. Let's look closely at each element:

DESCRIBE. In this phase you open your script by describing the situation that you have in mind. Your description should be as objective and specific as possible, so that your listener can understand what you're talking about.

EXPRESS. In this phase you express what you feel and think about whatever situation you have described. You can signal emotional expressions with phrases like *I feel that* or *I think that*. Here clarity and moderation work better than an emotional or sarcastic outburst.

Whenever possible, express your feelings about offensive behavior from a positive rather than a negative perspective. Negative expressions include phrases like *you make me angry* or *you're selfish and insensitive*. Though you may honestly feel that negative, you'll do better if you focus on positive, common goals.

SPECIFY. After describing the situation and expressing your feelings about it, ask explicitly for a specified behavior. Make your request reasonable and within the power of the other person to meet. For example, if your boss routinely gives you a lot of paper work near the end of the day, you would do better if you requested that you receive the paper work earlier in the day than if you requested that the boss do it. Because your appeal may rely partly on a charge of injustice and unfairness, you lose that advantage if you make unrealistic and unfair demands. Also, because we all resist change to a degree, limit your demand to the smallest change acceptable to you. If you have a big problem, break it into small pieces that you can address over a period of time.

Realize that your assertiveness about someone else's behavior may trigger a response from the other person for changes in your own behavior. There's nothing wrong with this. Indeed, successful outcomes often involve some give and take by both sides. For this reason analyze your request to see whether it might produce a counter-request. If it might, think about your possible responses to that counter-request. For example, if you ask the medical control director to change protocols to allow field personnel greater freedom of action, would you be asked to embark on an extensive training program first? You must ask yourself whether the costs of the training program exceed the gains achieved by the protocol changes. In this way you can determine whether you stand to lose more than you will gain by the exchange.

CONSEQUENCES. In this final phase of an assertive exchange you should clearly express the consequences of whatever agreement you wish to reach. This will be a reward for accepting the agreement or a penalty for not accepting it.

Rewards can be tangible or intangible. Sometimes a raise in pay is appropriate. But you have an almost unlimited number of other ways to express approval or show your appreciation to someone else: hugs, handshakes, pats on the back, extra days off, permission to work on new projects. The list is almost endless. Be creative.

Poor EMS managers use punishments more than rewards: threats of termination, written warnings, indifference to a person's needs, or criticism. Sometimes punishments are the only tactic that will work in a given situation. You should realize, however, that punishments always carry the risk that the other person will retaliate. As a result punishments and their repercussions can escalate minor annoyances into disasters. If you really must use the threat of punishment, make sure that you threaten only what you can deliver. Grandiose threats ruin your credibility and are ineffective.

In general you'll do better by stressing rewards over punishments. Always try using rewards first, resorting to threats of punishment only if all else fails.

Table 5–3 summarizes the key elements in developing an assertive message.

Scene 3 provided a good example of a well-executed DESC script. You might reread it and see how each of the four elements was used.

Use the DESC script as an outline when you need to be assertive. You'll find it helpful. The DESC script alone, however, won't be enough. What happens when someone interrupts you half-way through your description of the problem? How do you get back on track? Or worse yet, how do you handle another person who unexpectedly throws unjust or manipulative criticism at you? To cope with these tactics, you must learn another set of techniques developed by a noted authority on assertiveness, Manuel J. Smith.[8]

129

TABLE 5–3. DESC Outline Rules

DO	DON'T
Describe. Describe the other person's behavior objectively, using precise terms. If possible, describe a specified time, place, and frequency of action.	Make biased assessments. Use abstract terms or generalize.
Express. Express your feelings openly and calmly.	Pretend your feelings aren't affected. Unleash emotional outbursts.
Specify. Ask explicitly for a specific change in behavior. If possible, limit request to one or two small changes. Specify what you are willing to do to reach agreement.	Hint or imply that you'd like an unspecified change. Ask for large or multiple changes. Assume that only the other person has to change.
State consequences. Make the consequences explicit. Emphasize rewards that are desirable and reinforcing to the other person for change in the desired direction. Use punishments rarely. Select punishments of a magnitude that fit the crime and of a type that you are actually willing to carry out.	Discuss consequences in generalities or not at all. Use punishments as a first step. Select rewards that only you might find rewarding. Make exaggerated threats or threats you are unwilling to carry out.

Smith's techniques stem from three principles:

1. Don't reward people who try to manipulate you.
2. If you are attacked, don't counterattack.
3. If you have the proper training, you can handle any manipulative situation without becoming anxious or defensive.

To be an effective manager, it is important that you understand and use Smith's tools.

The first tool, called the *broken record*, helps you develop persistence. Many people intend to be assertive but become sidetracked and manipulated by others. Aggressive salesmen are notorious in this regard. Even though you may start with the best intentions, firmly convinced that you don't need what's being sold, somehow you end up the proud owner of the newest bandage on the market—an item destined to collect dust in the closet. The trick in these cases is to stick to your guns. All you need do is repeat the same simple phrase in response to each new approach that the other person takes. Suppose, for example, that a salesman walks into your office carrying a defibrillator. Using broken record, you might handle the situation in this way:

Salesman:	Here I have the greatest breakthrough in defibrillator technology, the Acme 4000DX. Because you're such a good customer, I thought I'd show it to you before any of my other accounts get a chance.
You:	Thanks for your courtesy, but we're not looking to buy any defibrillators right now.
Salesman:	Believe me, you won't want to pass up this opportunity. They've only given me a small quantity, and I'm sure they'll go fast. How many can I put you down for?
You:	Thanks, but we really don't need any.
Salesman:	Once these catch on, I expect the price to go right through the roof. It might pay to buy ahead. Tell me, what's the top energy of the defibrillator you've got now?
You:	Thanks, but we don't need any.
Salesman:	Tell you what. Just to get the ball rolling on these, I'll give you a 20 percent discount if you order one today. How does that compare to your usual price?
You:	Thanks, but we don't need any.
Salesman:	Of course, I'd be happy to leave one with you to evaluate free of charge. You see, I'm certain you'd love it. Where would you like me to put it?
You:	Thanks, but we don't need any.

After a while it becomes easier and easier to resist this type of manipulation. Eventually your message will get through.

The second technique, called *fogging*, consists of calmly accepting criticism, acknowledging that it may hold some truth. In some cases you can completely agree with manipulative criticism. For example:

> Critic: You're reading that magazine again.
>
> You: That's right; I *am* reading this magazine.

Following this type of reply, either your critic will express some *meaningful* criticism or drop the subject.

In other cases your critic doesn't state a case quite so factually. When the criticism takes the form of an opinion, you can assertively agree with the possibility that the opinion is accurate. For example,

> Critic: You're not very organized.
>
> You: Maybe I'm not very organized.

This approach withholds reward from your critic because you don't respond in a meaningful way to the meaningless generalization. Either the critic will specify some important examples or you will continue comfortably to slough off the manipulative ploys. This technique allows you to remain completely composed while giving up nothing.

Negative assertion, the third tool, is similar to fogging. With this skill you strongly agree with criticisms of yourself. You are neither angry nor apologetic when your flaws are pointed out; rather you agree with your critic that you're not perfect. For example,

> Critic: This report was due a week ago. You're late.
>
> You: You're absolutely right. I am late.

Such direct assertions of wrongdoing not only demonstrate your belief that even you can make a mistake, but they quickly exhaust your critic's anger so that the conversation can move constructively along, rather than harboring on blame.

Negative inquiry, the fourth tool, consists of probing your critic for further criticism. You can either use the criticism if it's constructive or exhaust it if it's manipulative. This encourages your critic to become more assertive. For example,

> Critic: Your EMTs don't present a neat appearance.
>
> You: What is it about our appearance that isn't neat?

Critic: Well, for one thing, look at your uniforms.

You: What is it about our uniforms that isn't neat?

Critic: Well, the color is fading and they're wrinkled.

You: Then it's the faded color and the wrinkles in our uniforms that detracts from our appearance?

Critic: Yes, for one thing.

You: Is there anything else that detracts from our appearance?

By focusing the conversation on yourself rather than your critic, you are less likely to elicit a defensive reaction. You break down defensive barriers when your words demonstrate a sincere interest in the critic's message. You must actively listen to what the other person is saying. This underscores the fact that it is just as important for both parties to hear each other as it is for both parties to present themselves clearly. The two go hand in hand.

Assertiveness, then, means many things. It means the freedom to express your feelings. It means taking account of the feelings of others. It means being open and honest with others and yourself, with sticking to your guns when you feel that it's right, with listening to others when they disagree with you. Developing assertiveness skills takes practice. Apply the skills outlined in this chapter every day, and your ability as a manager will improve.

Summary

Improving your ability to communicate is the first step in upgrading your directing skills. Many EMS problems arise from poor communication. EMS managers generally respond to these problems by communicating more often. To be an effective manager, however, you should strive for better communication. This requires that you be an active listener and an assertive speaker. The tools outlined in this chapter provide you with the fundamentals to improve your communication skills. If you practice these skills, you'll avoid many of the problems that plague EMS managers. Once you understand what skills you need to develop in order to improve your ability to communicate, you must learn how to apply those skills to a specialized form of EMS communication: negotiation.

6

Negotiating

I'm not a good negotiator because I'm not assertive enough. I don't give my needs a high priority. I guess that feeling stems from not feeling good about myself. I don't value my needs. So I give in too easily when I negotiate. I sabotage myself.
—STATE EMS OFFICIAL

Whenever two or more people confer to reach agreement, they negotiate. As an EMS manager, you negotiate daily. These negotiations range from simple problems, such as where to store a particular piece of equipment, to difficult problems, such as how to solve budget crises. The outcomes of these negotiations determine in large measure how successful you are in handling your responsibilities. For that reason you must possess effective negotiating skills.[1]

Negotiation is one of the most intensely studied areas of social interaction. Social psychology research includes more than a thousand studies conducted since 1960.[2] Obviously you don't have time to review all that material. You need the essentials, the principles that characterize effective negotiating, and some understanding of how you can apply those principles to your work.

Rule 1. In a successful negotiation everyone wins.

The inexperienced negotiator considers negotiation a game in which there is a definite winner and loser. In this view the goal of negotiation becomes defeating an opponent. This approach to negotiation is often ineffective; in general the results of negotiations between cooperative participants is more likely to produce a positive outcome than that between competitive participants. For this reason, you should consider negotiation a cooperative venture in which the goal is to reach an effective solution for all parties involved. This is particularly important in the case of repeated negotiations between the same two participants. If it is clear in one negotiation that one of the participants has won, then in the next negotiation the loser is likely to seek an unreasonable settlement in order to make the two parties even. This process of getting even is an ineffective pattern of negotiating.

"That's OK," you say, "but what happens if I view negotiation as a cooperative venture in which I want all parties to achieve an effective settlement, but my opposing negotiator views negotiation as a competition in which he wants everything and doesn't care about my needs? Do I give in?" Of course not—seeing negotiation as a cooperative venture does *not* mean that you become a patsy. You can be as tough as you need to be.

Rule 2. Time spent in preparation for negotiation is never wasted.

The successful negotiator's most important characteristic is that he does his homework. A good negotiator will not enter a negotiation blind. The outcome of a negotiation will depend largely on the thoroughness of preparations that you make before you negotiate. The thoroughness of your preparation should correspond to the difficulty and importance of the negotiation. You may want to begin preparing for important negotiations weeks or months before those negotiations are scheduled to start.

We spoke with the negotiators for a group of emergency physicians who were entering a hospital contract negotiation. The negotiation was with the board of directors of an urban teaching hospital that was experiencing a financial upheaval. Several new members of the board of directors believed that hospital-based physicians earned too much money. These board members were successful businessmen, and they were convinced that if they applied their business skills to negotiating new contracts, they could save the hospital a substantial amount of money. The board had appointed a negotiating committee, which first approached the pathologists. Several months of nerve-racking negotiations ensued. In the end the hospital negotiating team was successful in winning major financial concessions. Encouraged, the hospital negotiating team approached the radiologists. Again a prolonged negotiation ensued. The radiologists and the hospital negotiating team reached an impasse.

The emergency physician group watched this development with great concern; obviously they were next. Their contract still had several months to run, and they used that time to their advantage. They reviewed the techniques used in the previous two negotiations, held mock negotiations to develop counterarguments to those techniques, and determined their best negotiating stance. They investigated the opposing negotiating team in extreme detail. How had those negotiators behaved in previous negotiations away from the hospital? And perhaps most importantly, because the negotiators were claiming that the physicians made too much money, how much money did the opposing negotiators earn? (They earned considerably more than the physicians.) When the negotiations finally took place, the emergency physicians successfully negotiated the contract that they wanted.

Few negotiations will require this extent of preparation. But virtually all negotiations demand several basic steps.

The first thing that you must do is to determine who the players will be. Will you alone negotiate for your side or will you be a member of a team? In general, teams are more effective than individuals, because teams allow you to tap the expertise of others in areas where you might be weak. If you are a member of a team, who will be the team leader? What roles will the team members fulfill?

The second organizing step is to determine with whom you will be negotiating. For example, if the roof on your newly constructed ambulance garage is leaking, should you negotiate with just the roofing contractor or should you include the architect? In general you should make sure that all involved parties will be represented in the negotiation.

These two preparatory steps give you some understanding of the structure of the negotiation that you are entering. The next step in preparation is more difficult.

Rule 3. To be a successful negotiator, you must know your personal strengths and weaknesses.

Negotiations can be stressful and emotion-charged. Because most of us like to avoid situations like that, our attitude toward negotiations and our knowledge of our personal strengths and weaknesses can have an impact on our negotiations. Consider these comments from health-care providers taking a course on negotiation.

Director of
Nursing: I can't wait to get this over! I hate negotiations.

Instructor: Why is that?

Director of
Nursing: It all seems so dishonest. You say one thing. They say another. No one says what they really mean. It makes me uncomfortable. Maybe that's why I'm not any good at it.

And this:

EMS
Director: I don't mind negotiating. In fact, there are parts of it that I like a lot and do well. My problem is that when I negotiate a solution that I can accept, I get very anxious if I try for a better solution. I think "What's going to happen if I lose what I've

139

got?" Consequently I rarely do as well as I should when I negotiate. When I do try for a better solution, I get so nervous that I lose sleep. I say to myself, "Hey, it's not worth it!" I wish that I didn't feel that way. I wish that I were more detached.

The EMS director and the director of nursing highlight just two of the numerous emotional factors that can block effective negotiating. Let's examine three of the most significant blocks to effective negotiating: anxiety, barriers to creativity, and hidden assumptions.

ANXIETY. Do you become anxious when you negotiate? Think of the last time you tried to persuade a salesman to lower the price of a car or washing machine. Were your palms sweaty? Could you feel your pulse pounding? Anxiety is a key factor in negotiation.

How much anxiety and uncertainty can you stand? If you can tolerate a lot, chances are that negotiations don't bother you. If your tolerance is low, you will find negotiations unpleasant. You can take certain steps, however, to improve your negotiating ability. You should limit yourself to one negotiation at a time. Multiple concurrent negotiations can push your anxiety through the roof. You should continually narrow the areas of disagreement so that you have to deal with as little uncertainty as possible. You should negotiate for short periods to limit your exposure to anxiety. Take heart: For many people, negotiation-induced anxiety diminishes with experience.

BARRIERS TO CREATIVITY. Ask a group of first-graders how many of them can paint, and they all will probably say that they can. Ask a group of adults, and most will probably say that they don't have the talent. Are the adults stating a fact, or are they describing barriers to creativity that they have constructed around themselves? These barriers appear all the time in negotiations. How many times have you gone to a superior with a new solution to a problem, only to be told "This is the way we've always done it" or "I'm sure that won't work"?

To be an effective negotiator, you must consider all alternative solutions to a problem—the tried-and-true and the off-the-wall. The more solutions you investigate, the more likely you are to reach sound agreements during negotiation.

HIDDEN ASSUMPTIONS. We observed the negotiations of a private ambulance service in a small town. The town had a reputation for extreme financial conservatism. The ambulance service had begun as a basic-life-support unit but, during the initial contract, it upgraded the service to advanced life support. Because the costs increased when the service level was upgraded, it began losing money. EMS personnel in surrounding areas were convinced that the ambulance service would soon close because the town would never renegotiate the contract for the increased money that the ambulance needed. The ambulance service personnel, being new and inexperienced with the town's tight fiscal policy, held no such assumptions. They negotiated for a new contract and received it.

Hidden assumptions are always creeping into negotiations —"The manufacturer won't fix this under warranty...," "My medical director would never buy that...," "He told me that, he must have had a good reason...." Like barriers to creativity, hidden assumptions limit your chances of negotiating effective solutions to problems because they limit the number of solutions that you can investigate. Whenever you become aware that you are making an assumption, examine it to see whether there is any possibility that the assumption could be wrong. If there is, reject the assumption.

Rule 4. In a successful negotiation every participant has some needs met.

A negotiated settlement should meet as many of the needs of the negotiating parties as possible. An effective negotiator sees the issues being negotiated in terms of the personal, as well as institutional, needs of the opposing negotiator. The inexperienced negotiator frequently fails to appreciate the extensive variety of needs that motivate all of us and may place undue importance on satisfying only obvious needs. This is apparent in the often used and frequently unsuccessful patient-care argument. If you have been around EMS management for any time, you've experienced this approach. It consists of the manager's prefacing remarks with a statement like "All I care about is patient care," or "Someone is going to die if you don't...." Then the manager presents the details of the proposal. The manager's underlying assumption is that the opposing negotiator will respond to any plea that concerns patient care. Usually the opposing negotiator does not. The manager then reports that the failure occurred because the opposing negotiator "doesn't care about patients." In reality the manager's failure stems from two factors:

- Talking instead of listening. One key to effective negotiating is picking up the clues that the opposing negotiator reveals about important needs. Active listeners usually make able negotiators.
- Concentrating entirely on how the proposal satisfies the need to improve patient care. The manager pays little attention to the myriad of other needs of the opposing negotiator.

Needs fulfillment becomes the crux of successful, cooperative negotiations. Using Maslow's hierarchy of needs, you can predict which needs are likely to predominate in a particular situation.[3] Maslow postulates five levels of need:

- **Physiological Needs.** Primarily the homeostatic mechanisms of the body: maintaining blood pressure, blood sugar, acid-base balance, etc.
- **Need for Safety.** Security, stability, structure, and freedom from fear.
- **Need for Belonging.** Affection, family, positive responses from people in general.
- **Need for Esteem.** Achievement, status, recognition, and dignity.
- **Need for Self-actualization.** The desire to become everything that one is capable of becoming: A musician must make music; an artist must paint.

In Maslow's theory lower needs must be met before higher needs become significant. A hungry person, for example, will respond to food (physiologic need) more readily than to love (belongingness need). You will encounter similar responses in negotiations. An elected official, for example, is more likely to support an improvement in ambulance services if you show that it will aid in reelection (safety need) than if you argue that the service should be state-of-the-art (esteem need).

In analyzing yourself you must identify your own needs. What specific needs can be met by this negotiation? For example, if you are negotiating about the leak in the ambulance garage roof, your immediate need might be safety (prompt repair of the leak).

After identifying your general needs you must determine the specific goals that you expect to achieve in the negotiation. You should set your goals high because in general the more that you expect to achieve in a negotiation, the more you will achieve. A successful experience that we had illustrates this point. We purchased a small computer to assist us in data retrieval, word processing, and patient care. The computer developed the annoying habit of losing data from time to time. We returned the computer for repair. After it came back, we continued to use the computer even though the error occasionally recurred. After nine months we again returned the computer for repair. By this time the warranty had expired. We approached the negotiation about repair expecting that the manufacturer would repair the machine without charge, and after some discussion, the manufacturer did.

There is no place that hidden assumptions hinder your negotiating ability more than in your level of expectation. How often do you give up before you even start? "Of course, they wouldn't do that...." "We'll never get them to agree to...." Don't let these assumptions prevent you from asking for what you really want.

Rule 5. You never know until you ask.

Once you set your goals, stick to them. Success in negotiations is often linked to your maintaining a high level of expectations while your opponents lower theirs. For instance, in our example of the leaking garage roof, you might expect the contractor and the architect not only to repair the defective roof without cost but also to reimburse you for any water damage that occurred because of the faulty construction. Remember that the architect or the contractor will never agree to your goals unless you ask.

Next you should translate your goals into a range of acceptable settlements. Specifically you want to define your maximum and minimum acceptable settlements. The maximum acceptable settlement should be the best settlement that you can support by fact and logic. In cases of repeated negotiations between two parties you may also wish to limit the maximum acceptable settlement to the best settlement that you can obtain without the opposing negotiator feeling defeated. This avoids the problem of the opposing negotiator's trying to get even in future negotiations. The minimal acceptable settlement is the worst settlement that you will accept.

Once you define your limits of acceptable settlement, you

143

must plan the arguments that will support the goals that you have established. You should realize that when you present a series of arguments, your opponent is likely to remember best your first and last arguments and is less likely to remember those arguments in the middle. Therefore it is wise to present your best arguments first and last.

Another factor to consider is your bargaining power. Bargaining power is the ability not to give in during a negotiation. The party with the most bargaining power does not always achieve the best results in a negotiation; other factors, such as negotiating skill and personal needs, affect the settlement. Superior bargaining power, however, is a great advantage in a negotiation.

Rule 6. Whenever possible, negotiate from a position of strength.

You can assess bargaining power in a negotiation by asking three types of questions:

- What impact will it have on each party if you fail to agree during the negotiation?
- If you fail to agree, what sanctions can the opposing party bring against you, and what is the probability that the opposing party will do so?
- If you fail to agree, what sanctions can you bring against the opposing party? What are your costs of bringing those sanctions? What impact will those sanctions have on the opposing party?

EMS managers often incorrectly assess the bargaining power of the opposing negotiator. Bargaining power varies greatly from issue to issue and from one negotiation to the next.

In 1978, EMSS grants were running out in our region. Several other regions in our state were still receiving significant levels of federal grant money. Our local EMS region had not developed concrete plans for further funding. The private corporation that ran the state EMS system presented the region with the following proposal: The region would pay the corporation $90,000 per year in exchange for two regional coordinators. Furthermore, the corporation warned, failure to accept this plan would jeopardize all EMSS grants to the state. The region rejected the proposal for two reasons. First, because the EMS region no longer was receiving grant money, the threat would have no impact on the region. Second, the region concluded that it was highly unlikely the federal government would withhold major grant monies from the state over such a minor issue. In the end the region was correct. After a year of interim state support the region hired one coordinator for $20,000 dollars per year. No federal grants were terminated. This incident illustrates that a negotiator's bargaining power is subject to change over time and under differing circumstances.

Once a power relationship has been established in a negotiation, be careful that you don't take steps to reduce your power. We observed the negotiations between an emergency department director and a small rural hospital. While living in another state, the director made a verbal agreement of employment with the hospital. Before the contract was formally signed, the director quit his job and moved to the other state. This markedly diminished the director's negotiating strength because it eliminated the possibility that the director could stay at his old job if the new contract proved unacceptable. The hospital took advantage of the manager's weakened position by presenting a "corrected" contract that was markedly inferior to the original. The director, having no good option, signed the inferior contract.

As an EMS manager, you will negotiate in many situations where the opposing negotiator has the preponderance of power. The most frequent instance will be when you negotiate with your boss. If he disagrees with you, he can always fire you. You have no such direct power over him. In cases like this you can take several steps that will enhance your bargaining position even though your bargaining power is limited:

KNOWLEDGE. In general, the more that you know about the subject being negotiated, the better you'll do.

QUANTITATIVE ANALYSIS. Opponents often have a difficult time refuting supportable numbers.

COMPETITION. Opponents are more conciliatory when they face competition from outside sources. If you are negotiating with a vendor over an equipment purchase, for example, be sure that you shop around.

BUREAUCRACY. If it helps your negotiating position, you can say that rules and regulations prevent you from doing certain things. An experienced negotiator, however, will realize that those things are usually negotiable.

RELATIONS WITH YOUR OPPONENT. The better the relations between you and the opposing negotiator, the better your negotiating position is.

SUPPORT OF INFLUENTIAL PEOPLE. The support of influential people can enhance your bargaining position.

FORMING COALITIONS. Joining with other people or groups can improve your negotiating position and augment your power. This is a fairly common technique. We observed its use when a group of emergency department physicians joined together to form a multihospital group in a state where multihospital physician groups were rare. This step increased the physicians' negotiating power. The major risk of this approach is that it often threatens the opposing negotiator, who may retaliate by forming a coalition as well. That is exactly what happened. The hospital administrators met quietly behind closed doors and agreed not to deal with the new physician group. Thus the bargaining power gained by the first coalition was offset by the second.

When you understand your personal strengths and weaknesses, goals, range of acceptable settlements, and bargaining strength, you should turn your attention to the opposing negotiator. The analysis of your opponent proceeds along lines similar to the analysis of your own position. The importance of the negotiations will dictate the extent of your fact-finding search on your opponent. At the very least you should make an initial attempt at determining your opponent's organizational and personal needs. This is important for two reasons. First, this knowledge will assist you in directing your efforts to meet your own needs. For example, if your opponent's needs match yours identically in a certain area, you would waste time if you constructed lengthy arguments in support of your case in that area. Knowledge of your opponent's needs is also critical in achieving cooperative negotiations. Remember that it is important in the negotiation that your opponent's needs, as well as your own, be at least partially met.

Find out all that you can about your opponent's behavior in previous negotiations. Does the person usually set goals high or are they relatively modest? Anticipate what the opposition's arguments are likely to be in defense of goals, so that you can prepare counterarguments at this early stage. One significant error made by the inexperienced negotiator is to prepare arguments only in support of one's own position. This is just half the job; preparing counterarguments to your opponent's goals is the other half. Estimate your opponent's maximum and minimal acceptable settlements. If, for example, you are buying a new radio and the salesperson has quoted you a price, you know the maximally acceptable settlement. If you can determine the salesperson's cost for the radio, you have some idea of the other party's minimal acceptable settlement.

You should be able to determine your opponent's bargaining strength relative to yours. Review the same areas of potential strength that you did in assessing your own strength, only this time do it from your opponent's perspective.

Rule 7. Learn the opposing negotiator's deadline and make it work for you.

Deadline pressure is an effective force for compromise in a negotiation for three reasons:

- The heightened time pressure increases the importance of reaching agreement.
- Toughness requires time. As time pressure increases, tough negotiating stances are likely to be compromised.
- Under a heightened time pressure, concessions are unlikely to be perceived as a sign of weakness.

To be effective, you should learn the opposing negotiator's deadline and attempt to conduct negotiations as close to that deadline as possible. In that way the time pressure on the opposing negotiator is likely to induce adoption of a more conciliatory negotiating stance. From this you can see the advantage of having a deadline after the opposing negotiator's deadline or being so flexible as to have no deadline at all.

The corollary of this principle is that you should never reveal any deadline and should avoid answering questions such as "Oh, by the way, when are you going to need a final answer?"

Once you have examined your position and what you perceive to be your opponent's position, you should attempt to determine an agenda. You will need an agenda to ensure that you discuss all important issues; otherwise you may lose valuable time by negotiating over issues which are irrelevant. Agendas provide an organized means of discouraging the tendency to digress.

How you order the items on the agenda will vary depending on the negotiation. As a general rule top the list with issues where you feel your goals and your opponents goals are in concert. This approach will reduce your anxiety by quickly resolving many issues where there is little disagreement and will set a cooperative tone for the negotiations. It is much easier to maintain an established cooperative spirit than to try to create it after you and your opponent have dug in your heels on an issue that is difficult to resolve.

The final preparatory phase for negotiation is to test your position against what you perceive to be your opponent's position. Ask another member of your team or a coworker to act as your opponent; then test your position against this person. This process checks for gaps in your preparation. You will discover whether your goals and expectations are too high or too low, whether your position is supportable or weak, how well your arguments will stand up under fire, whether you fully understand your opponent's position, and how effectively you can control the negotiation.

When you complete the simulated negotiation, you are ready to begin formal negotiations. The first step is to agree on an agenda. Since you prepared an agenda in the preparatory phase, you can propose that your agenda be accepted. The second step is to determine the opposing negotiator's authority to commit to an agreement.

Rule 8. Whenever possible, negotiate with someone authorized to say yes.

It's common for a negotiator to consult with the board of directors or a senior official of the organization to receive final approval for a negotiated settlement. You must accept this. You should be careful, however, to avoid negotiating with someone who cannot or will not commit the organization on any significant issues or who has little or no room to compromise. If the opposing negotiator says, "My boss will never buy this," terminate the negotiation. Obviously the boss is the one who can commit the organization; you need to negotiate with that person. Negotiating with someone who can't say yes is a waste of time and can be a negotiating ploy designed to induce you to make initial concessions before being able to negotiate with someone in authority.

The third step in formal negotiations is to evaluate your opponent's proposal. When the opposing negotiator presents a proposal, you should not bargain but *listen*. Although you have tried to determine your opponent's needs and goals during prenegotiation, don't assume that you are clairvoyant.

By applying the techniques of active listening to your opponent's presentation you may learn new facts that could significantly alter your initial impression of your opponent's needs and goals. Use any or all techniques of active listening. Paraphrase your opponent's statements to ensure that you understand what is being said. Use reflection to ensure that you understand the feelings as well as the content of the message. Ask as many clarifying questions as necessary. Remember that questions can often determine the direction of a discussion. As such, the phrasing and timing of questions can have great significance. Your opponent can answer who, what, where, and when more easily than why and how. Choose your words carefully according to how extensive an answer you require. Timing of questions is also important. If you open a discussion with "What do you think of this plan?" you run the risk of freezing your opponent into an immovable position. Less direct approaches are usually advisable in the early stages of discussion.

Active listening requires attention to both verbal and nonverbal clues. You can learn a tremendous amount about your opponent by using your eyes as well as your ears. Watch body position, gestures, and facial expressions. The combination of your opponent's words and nonverbal clues reveals so much information that you might want to designate one member of your negotiating team strictly as a listener and observer.

When you present your proposal, make sure that it is as direct and fact-filled as possible. Don't be afraid to discuss both sides of an issue.

Rule 9. Emphasize mutual interest and cooperation.

The outcomes of cooperative negotiations tend to be better than those of competitive negotiations.

You want to determine two things from your opponent's initial presentation:

- What needs can you fulfill for the opposing negotiator?
- What is the other person's range of settlement?

Once you have answered these questions, you can begin negotiating for a settlement. As indicated by your agenda, start by discussing areas of agreement. This will lead to a positive feeling of cooperation. Deal with the areas of disagreement one at a time. If you can't reach agreement in one of the areas, lay it aside and come back to it later. Your goal in solving these disagreements should be to meet the needs of the opposing negotiator by proposing solutions as close to your maximum acceptable settlement as possible. Be sure that your proposals are supported by facts.

The give-and-take of offer and counteroffer will differ from negotiation to negotiation.

Rule 10. Have your opponent make the first concession or counteroffer.

This is not always possible. Experience shows, however, that the negotiator who makes the first concession is likely to be the one who concedes the most. Having made a concession, your opponent will expect you to reciprocate. When you do make concessions, concede minor points. When the midpoint between your offer and your opponent's offer is acceptable to you, consider offering to split the difference.

When you have settled all your differences, you should write a memorandum of understanding (MOU).[4] The MOU serves as a summary of your agreements and a basis for a future contract if you intend to write one. In less formal negotiations a written MOU may not be necessary. In those cases you should make a summarizing statement of the agreement as you understand it and see whether the opposing negotiator agrees.

Numerous tactics can be used in negotiations. You should be familiar with some of them.

Rule 11. Use threats rarely, in appropriate situations, and be prepared to back them up.

Inexperienced negotiators threaten too often. They may make threats because they don't know better techniques of reaching successful settlements. They may use threats if they have not prepared effective counterarguments before a negotiation. They may use threats inappropriately to win minor concessions. Often, if pressed, they do not back up the threats.

Threats can play a useful role in some negotiations.[5] First, you should use them only on questions of great importance, such as major quality-of-care issues. Second, you should use them only when positions have hardened in a negotiation where you have not achieved your minimal acceptable settlement. Third, you must be willing to carry out the threat if the settlement cannot be reached. Finally, you should use threats only when you are reasonably sure that the threat will work.

Threats are high-risk ventures, particularly when used during repeated negotiations between the same parties. In the first place, threats often induce the threatened negotiator to accept the losing portion of a win-lose settlement. This creates a competitive negotiation with its inherent ineffectiveness and problems of getting even. Second, threats generate hostility, which clouds future negotiation between the parties. Third, if you do not back up the threat, your credibility as a negotiator is lost.

We observed the negative nature of threats when the director of an ambulance service wanted to alter the work schedule so that his personnel could return to 24-hour shifts. He presented his reasons for the change, but his supervisor thought such a change unwise and turned down his request. Presented with the decision, the director stated that unless the change were made, he and at least half his crew would resign. Obviously the threat, if carried out, would present a significant problem. Nonetheless the supervisor stood firm and refused to alter the schedule. No one resigned. The ambulance director ceased being an effective negotiator after this incident.

On those occasions where threats are essential, remember the following three points:

- Threaten only what can be delivered. The threat should be large enough to cause disruption in the opposing organization. A threat is only too large if it interferes with credibility.

- Make definite preparations to carry out the threat. For example, if you threaten to quit your job, you might reinforce this by putting your house up for sale.

- Announce intentions to a third party. This gives the threat greater credibility.

Rule 12. Try to control the facts.

In a negotiation what is true depends on the negotiator's perceptions. Often one side believes that it has reached an agreement or defined a problem, only to find that the other side has no such belief. Defining issues, reaching solutions, and even determining truth thus become matters of negotiation. To be effective, you must control the "facts" of a negotiation or, at the very least, prevent the opposing negotiator from controlling them.

At 3 a.m. in a rural emergency department an automobile accident victim arrived. The patient had multiple injuries and blood in his urine. The practitioner on duty ordered an intravenous pyelogram (IVP). In order to perform the exam, however, a radiologist needed to be called. The radiologist considered the procedure inappropriate and called the emergency department director at home to complain.

Several days later the radiologist and emergency department director met to discuss the case and negotiate a policy concerning similar situations in the future. During the discussion the radiologist said, "Now I know I woke you from sleep, so you might not remember, but you very specifically said to me...." Whether the statement had been made was critical to the negotiation. In this case the radiologist was trying to substitute his perception of the events for fact. By doing so, he tried to increase the likelihood that the negotiated settlement that he favored would be accepted. By accepting the radiologist's version of the "facts," the ED director would relinquish substantial control in the negotiation. Instead of doing that, the director informed the radiologist that everyone has trouble remembering what is said at 3 a.m. Thus, the "facts" were open to negotiation.

You should be careful when the opposing negotiator says, "I have a very good memory and I remember that you specifically said...." or "I took notes of that meeting and you agreed to...." These are attempts by the opposing negotiator to define the facts in a negotiation. By doing so, the opposing negotiator attempts to increase the likelihood that a solution that he favors will be accepted. If your opponent's proposed version of the truth puts you at a disadvantage, refuse to accept it by saying: "I don't recall saying that..." or "I don't have any notes of agreeing to that...."

Another element in controlling "facts" is that you should never let the opposing negotiator write the sole memorandum of understanding (MOU). An effective opposing negotiator will insist on writing the MOU in order to slant the "facts" of the agreement subtly. If a summary is to be written, you should write it. If that is unacceptable to the opposing negotiator, then both negotiators should write MOUs with the final product being negotiated from the two summaries.

Summary

Like communication, negotiation is a key managerial skill for directing your service and its personnel. Although negotiation is a skill that must be developed through practice, understanding and applying the 12 basic rules of negotiation that you learned in this chapter will give you a head start over other EMS managers. As your skill as a negotiator increases, you'll become a more successful manager. Your managerial skills will improve even further if you can effectively apply a third directing skill, delegation, which we will discuss in Chapter 7.

7

Learning to delegate

Do you want to know how it really works? In our service, if you want something done right, you do it yourself. I'll bet almost everyone in this room would say the same thing about their service.
—EMT, ATTENDING MANAGEMENT TRAINING SEMINAR IN HOPES OF BEING PROMOTED TO SUPERVISOR

How many times have you heard the expression, "If you want
something done right, do it yourself"? Most EMS systems operate under that principle. If you want to be an effective EMS
manager, however, you must delegate competently whenever
possible. Otherwise you'll find your time constantly absorbed by
tasks that could be done better by someone else. You must
change the motto to "If you want something done right, find the
right person to do it."

This chapter will show you how to delegate effectively. What
is *delegation*? Simply defined, *delegation* is giving people things
to do. Remember the last time your supervisor asked you to do
something that he or she could have done: That's delegation.
Delegation has many benefits, which we'll examine in this chapter. Unfortunately, despite these benefits, many EMS managers
have a difficult time delegating effectively. It's important that
you understand why this is, so that you can avoid the same trap.

The delegation process

Let's begin our examination by discussing the three features that
characterize delegation:[1]

1. A manager assigns certain duties to a subordinate.

2. A manager grants authority to a subordinate to carry out
   those duties.

3. A subordinate accepts the responsibility of performing
   those duties for a manager.

Assigning duties

What types of duties should you delegate? We'll touch on this in
greater depth later, when we distinguish between managing and
doing. For now, though, realize that delegation should proceed
directly from an analysis of the work goals that you determined
for yourself in Chapter 1. As you subdivide your goals into
specific activities, consider any of the following activities as
suitable for delegating:

1. Matters that continually recur.

2. Minor decisions made frequently.

157

3. Time-consuming jobs. (These are not always routine. For example, not everyone can handle the responsibility of training new workers, but probably someone in your department would be excellent at it.)

4. Areas of responsibility that you consider low priority.

5. Jobs that can be performed better by someone other than you.

6. Job details that you dislike. (There's nothing wrong with making your work more enjoyable, particularly if someone else might enjoy jobs that you find disagreeable.)

7. Jobs that can be completed on a more timely basis by someone else, particularly where timeliness is important.

8. Jobs that will help develop a subordinate. (Delegating tasks outside an employee's normal area of expertise will encourage that employee to grow.)

Granting authority

The second feature of delegation is that the manager must grant authority to a subordinate. Granting authority gives the subordinate the required power to carry out the responsibility. For example, if you delegate to an EMT shift supervisor the responsibility to ensure that the second ambulance shift is adequately covered, you must grant the authority to establish a schedule, alter EMTs' shifts to meet the schedule, and take appropriate action if an EMT misses a shift.

In general, you should delegate to your subordinate enough authority to carry out the delegated task. You should define authority as clearly as possible when you delegate. Vagueness in level of authority can lead to friction within an organization. A subordinate can get into trouble when limits of authority are so vague that the person either goes far beyond the appropriate sphere of action or fails to exercise the necessary initiative. Written job descriptions, policies, and procedures should indicate the authority of each member of an organization. In the purchasing area, for example, you might delegate to a subordinate the authority to initiate expenditures for individual items costing up to $200, with your approval required on purchases above this limit. Such specific limitations offer a measure of security to those delegated the responsibility to complete a task.

Accepting responsibility

The third common feature of delegation is the acceptance of an obligation by a subordinate. If you delegate a task to someone, that person must agree to do it. By taking the personal responsibility for completing a task, your subordinate can't pass the buck.

In general your subordinates are more likely to welcome delegation when you clearly explain your expectations for performance. You should document this in the duties and standards in the employee's job description in accordance with the recommendations in Chapter 3.

Benefits of delegation

At this point you might ask: Why would anyone agree to accept a delegated task? Our experience has shown that this is a concern of many EMS managers. In point of fact, however, EMS personnel tend to welcome additional delegated responsibility. If you think back to our discussion of managing for motivation in Chapter 2, you'll remember the findings of Herzberg and his associates. They found that the five key employee motivators were recognition, responsibility, achievement, the work itself, and advancement. Delegation, more than any other management tool, enables you to tap into these powerful motivating forces. Here's why:

1. If you delegate an important task to an employee based on the quality of his or her previous work, you have granted *recognition* of performance.

2. In delegating the new task you increase the employee's *responsibility*.

3. With increased responsibility the employee can experience a greater sense of *achievement*.

4. If you carefully choose which tasks to delegate to an employee based on your knowledge of the person's interests, you encourage greater employee satisfaction in *the work itself*.

5. If the new task changes the employee's job description enough to result in a new title or a higher level in your job grading system, you have granted *advancement* to the employee.

159

No other single management act can satisfy all the key employee motivators as effectively. As a result you should delegate to appropriate employees whenever possible.

As a delegating manager, you also benefit from delegation. Above all else, *delegation extends results from what you can do to what you can control.*

Successful delegation can double or triple your output as soon as you begin to achieve your results through the multiplied efforts of others. Delegation also releases some of your time for more important work. Even if you feel that you can perform a job better than your subordinates, the choice is not between the quality of your work versus theirs. The real choice depends on how you answer the question, *What is the best use of my time right now?*

In answering, you should realize that while many of your subordinates can perform parts of your job, only you can *plan, organize, direct,* and *control.* These tasks are the core of managing in EMS and should be top priority.

Managing vs. doing

If you are to manage effectively, you must be able to identify what a management task is. Many EMS managers have jobs that combine managing and doing. A physician-manager may combine seeing patients in an emergency department with managing. An EMT-manager may combine making ambulance runs with being a manager. These combinations work if you have enough time to do all that is expected of you. In most cases, however, you don't have enough time. In general, while you can delegate tasks that involve doing, you can't delegate tasks that involve managing. When your time is severely limited, you should seriously question yourself if you are spending your time on any activity that does not fall into one of the four management areas.

To illustrate the difference between managing and doing, we have prepared an exercise. Examine the following list of tasks and identify which ones are managing tasks and which ones are doing tasks:

1. Seeing a salesman who has called on you with a new monitor-defibrillator
2. Deciding whether to add a clerical position
3. Deciding what the expense budget will be for next year

4. Giving a talk to the local chamber of commerce about your EMS system

5. Explaining to one of your employees reasons for a raise

6. Interviewing a prospective employee referred to you by a friend

7. Reviewing your monthly expense budget

8. Attending a seminar to learn the latest techniques in intubation

TASK 1. Seeing a salesman who called on you is doing. You could delegate this job to someone else. If your organization is large enough to have a full-time purchasing agent, this individual should be screening salesmen. If you have no such individual, you can delegate this responsibility to one of your subordinates. Your own involvement in purchasing should be limited to a few specific areas. First, you must understand the fundamentals of purchasing that we discussed in Chapter 4 so that you can train one of your personnel to handle this function. Training falls within the organizing functions of management. (In some cases you can delegate it by training a trainer.) Second, you should determine the major pieces of equipment to be purchased; you resolved this during your formulation of a capital budget. (We discussed this in Chapter 4.) Budgeting, like training, is an organizing function. Third, you monitor your employee's purchasing performance through the use of regular budget reports. (We'll discuss this further in Chapter 10.) Monitoring your service's finances and appraising your employee's performance are controlling functions.

TASK 2. Deciding whether to add a clerical position is managing. Determining the staffing levels necessary to perform the organization's work (work measurement) is one of the organizing functions of a manager. You should not delegate this responsibility to anyone else.

TASK 3. Deciding what the expense budget will be is managing. When you establish a budget level, you are organizing—allocating your financial resources for a future period. You should not delegate this responsibility to anyone else.

TASK 4. Giving a talk to the local chamber of commerce is doing. It doesn't qualify as planning, organizing, directing, or controlling. Rather it is public relations and is often best performed by someone specifically responsible for this function. If an outside group asks you to speak, you should refer this request to that individual unless there are compelling reasons why you would be the only one able to speak.

TASK 5. Explaining to an employee reasons for a raise is managing. You are taking an opportunity to grant recognition to your staff. This is a powerful motivating and directing force. You should not delegate this task to anyone else.

TASK 6. Interviewing a prospective employee referred to you by a friend is doing. Someone else could handle this job. If your organization is large enough to justify a full-time personnel director, this individual should be screening applicants. If you have no such individual, you can delegate this responsibility to one of your subordinates. Your involvement in employment should be limited to a few specific areas. First, you should be responsible for determining your staffing levels (organizing). Second, you should provide the individual actually doing the interviewing with guidelines as to the qualifications of the individual whom you are seeking (organizing). Third, you should reserve the right of final approval before an applicant is hired (controlling). If at all possible, you should delegate the tedious process of reviewing all interested applicants to someone else.

TASK 7. Reviewing your monthly expense budget is managing. Establishing a budget for a future time period is organizing; comparing that budget to actual expenses is controlling. If actual expenses differ significantly from the budget, you can take appropriate corrective action. You should not delegate this responsibility to anyone else.

TASK 8. Attending a seminar to learn the latest techniques in intubation can be either doing or managing, depending on how you plan to use the information that you learn. If you are learning to improve your personal skills, you are doing. If you are learning in order to reassess the practices of your service with the possible reorganization of resources in mind, you are managing. This highlights one of the reasons why you should define your expectations of educational programs before you enroll. Be sure that such programs are consistent with your overall goals, because they consume large blocks of your time.

How did your answers compare to ours? If you remember anything from this exercise, it should be this: You must constantly evaluate your work to ensure that you are performing all necessary management functions. You should delegate doing functions whenever possible.

The principle of decision level

Delegation leads to better decision making, because it maintains a principle known as decision level.[2] This principle states:

You should delegate decisions to the lowest level where relevant facts and sound judgment are available.

This principle disputes the notion that the higher the level at which a decision is made, the better the quality of the decision. Policy decisions may need to be made at top levels; operating decisions, however, are often better made at lower levels in the organization where more complete facts and special expertise are available.

Barriers to delegation

Given the many benefits afforded by delegation, why is this tool used so sparingly? Many barriers block an expanded use of delegation, some stemming from the delegator and some from the subordinate.[3]

Perfectionism

Some EMS managers fail to delegate even the simplest tasks because they feel that they can do the job better themselves. Perfectionists in particular have problems if things aren't done just the way they want. Other EMS managers, although able to delegate the basic elements of a job, still feel an insatiable desire to

163

know all the details or keep a finger (or even a whole hand) in every pie. These attitudes instill insecurity in subordinates and waste time that should be devoted to higher level managerial functions.

Fear

Many EMS managers fail to delegate from fear. Perhaps you lack confidence in your subordinates and fear that they will make major mistakes in anything that you delegate to them. You need not fear this if you select competent subordinates, carefully train them, and provide control mechanisms to ensure that tasks are completed as planned.

Some EMS managers fear that by delegating they will lose some of their responsibility; perhaps they even threaten their own job security. A nurse summed up this feeling best by saying, "If I delegated all the things I could, I wouldn't have a job left." This fear is a major barrier to delegation. In part this fear stems from a misconception of what happens to responsibility when you delegate. Some managers believe that once they have delegated a duty, they no longer have any obligation for its accomplishment. That is not true. Even though you have delegated the responsibility to complete a task to a subordinate, you still are responsible to your supervisor for the task's completion. The organizational chain of command must remain intact. As such, you should not fear a loss of responsibility when you delegate. You couldn't lose that responsibility even if you wanted.

Another barrier is a manager's fear that employees will resent delegated duties as an additional burden on their workload. This assumption is clearly refuted by research correlating the degree of delegation employed by managers with ratings of the managers by their employees; managers who delegate frequently are more highly rated.[4] Remember our earlier discussion: Delegation motivates employees.

The greatest fear in delegating is deciding how to utilize the free time that you gain. This is particularly true if you have been promoted from the ranks of your department without any management training. Suppose that you are an EMT who has recently assumed the responsibility for managing your service. You may find yourself drifting back into your old job duties, like inspecting ambulances each morning to ensure completeness of supplies. You are already competent in these areas; in fact you probably excel at them—that's why you were promoted to a managerial position. These old jobs offer you security if you are uncomfortable with management responsibility, but they are an inappropriate use of your time in your new role.

Lack of delegating skills

Some EMS managers fail at delegation because they lack certain skills. For example, effective delegation requires that the manager plan far enough ahead to be able to train a subordinate to perform the necessary tasks. An EMS manager who promotes crisis management or who never plans a work schedule will fail to provide adequate training, and that manager's efforts at delegation will not be successful.

EMS managers must also know how to balance workloads. Remember:

It does no good to transfer duties from an overworked you to an overworked somebody else.

You must choose someone who has the time to handle the assignment.

A good delegator must also clearly explain what is expected of a subordinate. Poor teaching techniques will leave the employee confused and incapable of handling the assigned duties. This situation often arises when an EMS manager dislikes an activity and has never taken the time to learn how to perform it properly. This manager hopes to avoid it by handing it over to a subordinate. This situation really isn't delegation; it's dumping—one infallible way to turn off an employee to real delegation in the future.

Lack of control

Another barrier exists when the EMS manager doesn't establish effective control over a delegated situation. When you delegate a duty, you have actually substituted one job for another.[5] Although you no longer perform the delegated duty, you are now responsible for controlling somebody else doing the work. You must establish a workable control mechanism so that you can identify and correct small problems before they develop into larger ones. (We'll discuss this further in Chapter 9.)

Resistance by subordinates

Managers aren't the only source of barriers to delegation; subordinates can create roadblocks. Although delegation serves as a strong motivator for most people, some employees perceive a risk in added responsibility. They may fear making mistakes because they lack self-confidence. One technique for overcoming this is to provide experiences with increasingly difficult problems. The employees will slowly realize their own potential.

Some employees will resist delegation if they feel that they lack the necessary information and resources to accomplish the job successfully. As said earlier, you should state the employee's authority as clearly as possible and try to match it closely to the job's responsibility.

Reverse delegation

Any of these barriers can lead to reverse delegation, where a decision that was delegated to an employee is inappropriately returned to the manager.[6] There is nothing wrong with coaching and supporting your subordinates. A problem arises, however, when you actually assume responsibility for a task previously delegated. You must guard against doing this. Before you conclude a meeting in which you've discussed a delegated responsibility with a subordinate, ask yourself: Does the responsibility still rest with the subordinate? Be sure that the next move still remains with the subordinate. If the ball has somehow worked its way back into your court, you're a victim of reverse delegation. When reverse delegation occurs, analyze the situation and take corrective action to reestablish responsibility with the subordinate.

Another way that you encourage reverse delegation is by restricting a subordinate's authority so tightly that you must be consulted on every minor detail. In general, you can establish six levels of delegated authority:

1.   Don't do anything until I tell you.
2.   Ask me what to do, then act.
3.   Recommend a course of action and we'll discuss it. Then act in accordance with the conclusions.
4.   Act, but advise me at once.

5. Act on your own, then routinely report to me.
6. Act on your own.

To limit reverse delegation, you should avoid the use of levels one and two. The greater the level of delegated authority, the less likely reverse delegation will occur.

The delegation work sheet

Examine the delegation work sheet on the following page. This work sheet has proved an effective tool in EMS management. It integrates many of the key elements covered in this chapter and serves as a useful guide when you are contemplating a delegation of duty.

Summary

Delegation is the third key skill in directing your personnel. Successful delegation motivates your employees and extends results from what you can do to what you can control. It emphasizes a shifting of your priorities away from routine tasks toward the managerial functions of planning, organizing, directing, and controlling. In order to realize these benefits, you must recognize that barriers can block the effective use of delegation. You must identify and eliminate these barriers if you are to be successful.

Communication, negotiation, and delegation form the core of what you need to know to direct your EMS personnel. However, because EMS is a rapidly changing field, you need one additional skill: directing change.

EMS DELEGATION WORK SHEET

1. Results

    What are the expected results of this delegation?

2. Balancing Work Loads

    To whom are you delegating?

    What duties does that person have?

    How many hours will this new task require?

    Can the person handle the new load?

3. Authority

    What authority will the person need to achieve the expected results?

4. Training

    How will you train this person?

5. Control

    How will you monitor this delegation to ensure that you achieve the results that you expect?

Directing change

8

Whenever we tried to institute change, we met a wall of resistance. Even after all these years, I don't really understand why that resistance occurred. Maybe it has something to do with me. It was particularly frustrating because the changes we proposed proved to be right. And a few years after we proposed the changes, those people who strongly opposed us turned around and instituted the same changes we had proposed.

—EMS DIRECTOR

As EMS managers, we are constantly managing change. Sometimes through luck or skill we can make change occur smoothly. But new programs, no matter how well-conceived and important, always seem to make someone angry or uncomfortable. Just when you think that you've covered all bases before introducing something new, someone whom you hadn't considered storms into your office, irate over your program. It's frustrating to be battling continual resistance to positive, new programs that you're trying to introduce. When things go sour, you feel, "Doesn't anyone else care about this place?"

We spoke with the medical director for an active, nonprofit ambulance service. He was intelligent, highly motivated, and convinced that training his personnel to the paramedic level was important for high-quality prehospital care. The EMTs in the ambulance service were also convinced of the importance of training; many of them looked forward to upgrading their skills. The town would benefit from the advanced training. On the surface everything appeared promising, and training went forward. We talked with the director midway through the training course and complimented him on his efforts. "It's nice to hear something positive for a change," he said. "Maybe I'm just becoming defensive, but it seems that so many people are shooting arrows at me right now, I don't know which way to duck. It's becoming frustrating." He had encountered tremendous resistance while introducing a program that everyone had wanted. What went wrong?

In this chapter you'll learn the answer by examining the nature of tasks, resistance to change, and effective managerial strategies to direct change.[1]

The nature of tasks

The process of introducing and implementing a new program can seem chaotic and confusing. If you step back and study the nature of tasks, however, you will find that certain consistent facts apply to all tasks.[2] The first major principle that you must understand is this:

All tasks share the same four phases from beginning to end.

These phases are the introductory phase, the resistance phase, the productive phase, and the termination phase.

PHASE 1: THE INTRODUCTORY PHASE. This is the euphoric phase that we all enjoy. In the preceding example it was the period when the ambulance service's medical director said, "Let's upgrade the service to the paramedic level." He was greeted by cheers and "What a great idea!" The introductory phase is a period of great excitement—new and interesting things are about to happen. As a manager, you are likely to be swept up with the excitement during this period; after all, everyone is telling you what a great idea you've had. You begin to believe what you're being told and think that you're really a terrific leader. During the excitement you never ask yourself, "If this is such a great idea, why is it no one has done it before me?" Such doubts rarely arise. A new crusade is about to begin and you are going to lead it.

PHASE 2: THE RESISTANCE PHASE. Once the proposed idea sinks in, people begin to see its true impact. The proposed change will disrupt the status quo and will create real or imagined hardships. People evaluate your "great idea" in terms of the changes that it will require them to make. In a short period you go from the hero leading your troops into the crusade to the villain making a number of unwarranted changes. This is a period of working through resistance to change. Expect your leadership to be questioned. The director in the example aptly described the feeling of the resistance phase when he said "...so many people are shooting arrows at me right now, I don't know which way to duck." During the resistance phase it is easy to lose sight of the reasons why you undertook the change in the first place.

PHASE 3: THE PRODUCTIVE PHASE. Assuming that you work through the resistance phase, you enter the productive phase, where the group actually accomplishes the intended task. If you handled the resistance phase adequately, people begin to pull together, submerging their reservations. The group begins to see success and that success is reinforcing. In the preceding example the productive phase is the period when the paramedic training actually takes place—the courses start, the protocols are written, licensing details are completed.

PHASE 4: THE TERMINATION PHASE. One fine day the newly trained paramedics hit the streets. The staff members can enjoy the benefits of their labor. For you as a manager, it's a time to reexamine the total picture. Have all the goals been met? Have any important details been overlooked? Have you designed effective controls to ensure continued success? It's also a time to savor your accomplishment; as we said in Chapter 2, the feeling of closure is important. Whenever possible, stop to appreciate when you have completed a task.

That's the way tasks work. Of course, there are minor differences from time to time. Resistance may be a major problem on a large, controversial task but only a minor problem on a small task when everyone is united. In every new task that you begin, however, realize that to be successful you must pass through all four phases.

You can remove much of the mystery from effective leadership if you realize that

The resistance phase is the most constant and predictable obstacle to successful task completion.

If you want to complete difficult tasks, you must learn to predict and reduce the severity of the resistance phase.

Resistance to change

You should realize that normal, healthy people resist change. This explains why so many people shoot arrows at you when you begin to implement changes. There are three major reasons why healthy people resist change.

1. Fear of losing something of value

As a manager, you must not overlook the negative consequences of a proposed change. Realize that although change may not have negative consequences for you, it may for your personnel.

Manager: This new schedule is going to save us a lot of money. That should help make our service more viable in these hard times and your job will be more secure.

173

Paramedic:	Yeh, I want my job secure. But you've got me working two nights, then a 3 to 11, then a day, then two nights. My wife's going to have a fit.
Manager:	I'm sure that you can work it out.

It's perfectly reasonable for the paramedic to resist your proposed change, regardless of the money that it will save and the job security that it will create. It steals time that he can spend with his family. Change often has such negative consequences on personnel. We overlook those consequences if we don't take the time to elicit them. During the euphoria of the introductory phase it's much easier to assume that you're going to have clear sailing than it is to dig out all the reasons why you might not.

2. Misunderstanding of the change and its implications

As an EMS manager, when you propose a change, you have a fair idea of what the change involves. You must accurately communicate this to your employees. If you don't, your personnel may receive a distorted message. As you learned in Chapter 5 on "Improving Your Ability to Communicate," people will distort messages because of their existing attitudes. Consequently, when change threatens people who already feel insecure, they may distort the message into something even more threatening. We experienced problems, for example, when we tried to integrate our ambulance service with the emergency department. Although this change was threatening to both the ambulance service and the emergency department personnel, we ignored clues about potential resistance. As a result, when we tried to integrate the two services, we failed. We assembled our department personnel for a meeting, which went like this:

EMS Director:	I realize that this isn't working out very well. I'm wondering if there is anything we can do to make it work better.
(Silence)	
EMS Director:	I had hoped that we could all work together.
(Long silence)	
Nurses' Aide:	Are we going to lose our jobs?

174

That's when the resistance finally surfaced. The staff believed that we planned to replace present employees with EMTs. Although we had never planned to do that, a portion of the serious resistance stemmed from this misunderstanding.

3. Belief that the change does not make sense for the service

As an EMS manager, you should have a vision of what you want your service to become. Don't expect all your personnel to accept your viewpoint, however. When we tried to upgrade our ambulance service training level, for example, we met resistance stemming from the decision to employ only higher skilled personnel.

EMS Director:	That means that all of you must upgrade your skills to continue working here.
EMT:	I think that's a bad idea.
EMS Director:	Why?
EMT:	For one thing, it's going to be a lot more difficult to replace someone.

Of course, the EMT was right. It was going to be much more difficult to replace people. Although we had considered this, we believed that the advantages gained by improved care outweighed the disadvantage of less staffing flexibility. The EMT disagreed. As an EMS manager, you should not assume that everyone shares your perspective of what is best for the service. Resistance often occurs because your personnel honestly do not believe that your change makes sense for the service.

Even though resistance to change may be a natural occurrence, you must control that resistance so that your service's tasks can move forward.

The sooner you uncover a project's resistance, the better.

During the exuberant introductory phase you may tend to ignore potential resistance. Recognize this blindspot. If your personnel say, "That's a good idea, but ... , " be careful not to pass off their comments lightly with general statements like "Oh, we'll take care of that when the time comes." Instead of acting like a cheerleader and whipping up enthusiasm for your new project, you should bring forth criticism. Our EMS director in the first example would have done better if he had said at the outset, "I know that everybody might think going to the paramedic level is a good idea, but can anyone think of reasons why it might *not* be smart or of someone who might become upset about it?"

If you elicit resistance early in a project, you can plan an approach to it.

Predicted resistance is easier to handle than resistance that comes as a surprise.

Resistance that comes as a surprise is both difficult to handle and emotionally stressful. As a result you should ask your staff the following:

- Who is likely to oppose the proposed change?
- Why are they likely to oppose it?
- How and when will they express their resistance?

Once you have determined the answers to these questions, you can plan your approach to handling resistance. Although you can never predict all resistance, this approach enables you to predict much of it.[3]

Adjust the speed of your project to the amount of resistance that you expect.

When you encounter significant resistance, slow your project so that you can deal with the resistance and form a coalition of the project's supporters. This may be impossible if you have an externally controlled deadline by which you must complete the project. In the absence of such a deadline, however, make sure that you consider resistance when you develop a timetable.

Once you have identified who is likely to resist your proposed change and when and how they are going to express that resistance, select the tools that you are going to use to deal with the situation. There are five commonly used tools:

1. **Education and Communication.** Because a misunderstanding of the change and its implications is a major cause of resistance, one method of countering resistance is through education and communication. Active listening skills are helpful here. You must understand the ex-

act problems and misunderstandings that people have about your proposed change. A good education program at the outset can help limit misunderstandings.

2. **Participation and Involvement.** Whenever possible, present only the general outline of a proposed change. Let your subordinates fill in the details. Participation and involvement are critical in many projects. Personnel support ideas more when the ideas are their own. Allow them the opportunity to propose changes whenever possible.

3. **Facilitation and Support.** Every change causes stress and anxiety. Your support during this period is helpful to your personnel. Accordingly you must be visible and available. Don't propose a change and then hide in your office to work on it. Spend time with the people whom the change will affect.

4. **Negotiation and Agreement.** One cause of resistance is a desire not to lose something of value. If a proposed change will mean that certain people will lose out, try to negotiate acceptable settlements.

5. **Coercion.** EMS managers use coercion and threats more than they should. Although coercion may be helpful in cases where speed is important, recognize that it doesn't effectively deal with resistance over the long run. As a result you can expect resistance to resurface at a later time.

Developing and using your leadership strength

In the previous section you've learned the techniques for successfully completing tasks that involve change. Applying these techniques will enable you to handle the many changes that confront you as an EMS manager. Improving your strength as a leader will also help.[4,5]

In Chapters 5, 6, and 7 you learned directing techniques that will dramatically increase your leadership ability. Listening well, asserting yourself, negotiating competently, and delegating frequently will make you a better leader. In addition to those methods there are three additional steps you can take:

1. Control tangible resources.

We spoke with the vice president of a successful emergency medicine group. This group, which began as three physicians running one emergency department, has grown to a multistate organization that owns and manages freestanding clinics and hospitals. We asked the vice president what was the single most important step for a new EMS manager. He said: "Control the money. If you control the money, everything else will follow."

Budgets, employees, buildings, and equipment are the tangible resources that the manager can control. By controlling those resources an EMS manager increases leadership strength.

2. Control information and information channels.

In complex systems information is essential for rational problem solving. In a regional EMS system the regional manager often has strength because of the ability to provide services with scarce information.

3. Establish favorable relationships.

You can increase your leadership strength by establishing favorable relationships with your personnel. As a manager, you must provide other people with a reason for letting you decide something.

You establish favorable relationships when others feel obligated to you. Doing favors for your subordinates can often instill in them a sense of obligation. Few people form friendships or perform favors solely to create a sense of obligation; most of us would see this as dishonest and manipulative. However, honest kindness and consideration can build loyalty in your personnel, which will increase your leadership strength.

A second method of establishing favorable relationships is to develop your professional reputation. Achievements often confer leadership strength; the larger and more visible the achievement, the greater the strength it is likely to generate. For the EMS manager, writing articles for scientific journals, appearing on television or in the newspaper, and winning awards can be means to increase leadership strength.

A third method is to encourage your subordinates to identify with you. The more a subordinate identifies with the manager, the more likely the subordinate is to support the manager's decisions. Consider who would be supported more in a service where all the members worked their way up: a manager who progressed through the ranks or one brought in from the outside? Identification can enhance your leadership strength; emphasize your common bond with your subordinates. Make your successes your personnel's successes.

Once you have developed your leadership strength, you must use it carefully. In general you can use it either directly or indirectly. There are two direct ways:

1. **Commands.** If you have power over an individual, you can directly command that person to behave in a particular way. The chief advantage of this approach is clarity and speed. For example, you might tell an EMT, "Look, I'm in charge here, and I want you to be at that meeting this afternoon." Provided you have power over the EMT, you can force him to attend the meeting. The disadvantage of this approach is that EMS personnel don't like to be ordered around. If you use this approach exclusively, you'll generate hostility and in time your leadership strength will diminish.

2. **Persuasion.** The key to persuasion lies in using information that will affect another person's interests and goals. A persuasive manager convinces employees that some action (which the manager wants) is in their best interest, while other actions are not. The key here is to understand your staff's interests and tailor the proposed change to meet those interests. Using active listening techniques—enabling you to elicit the needs of your employees—is the first step. Then you can alter the nature of the change so that it can meet those needs.

You can use your leadership strength indirectly in two ways:

1. **Communicating through others.** Suppose that one of your personnel won't listen to you. You might consider speaking to a third party who has influence over that person. Although this approach can work, those managers who become labeled as manipulators are rarely successful.

2. **Restructuring the environment.** Realize that the forces that surround a person have a great impact on personal

behavior. The more of those forces that you control, the greater the likelihood that you can direct a person's behavior. You can restructure the environment by altering job descriptions, working conditions, policies, and merit systems. This approach has several advantages. First, it rarely involves a direct confrontation of employees. Second, once made, the change operates independently of the manager. Third, by changing the organizational rules, employees change their behavior on their own initiative without being told. Such changes are likely to stick.

Summary

If you want to succeed in EMS, you must direct change effectively. You must realize that resistance to change is a natural phenomenon. By applying the techniques outlined in this chapter you can manage that resistance so that your service is able to complete even difficult tasks. In the long run you'll be able to direct change better if you increase your leadership strength. By developing favorable relationships, emphasizing your common bond with your personnel, and sharing your achievements, your leadership strength will increase. You must be subtle in how you use that strength, however. You should emphasize persuasion rather than commands, and restructuring the environment rather than confrontation.

By applying the skills that you've learned in Section III, you will be able to direct your EMS personnel effectively to achieve your service's objectives. Your job as a manager isn't over at this point, however. You must be sure that your objectives are achieved by developing control mechanisms. These control mechanisms can alert you to potential problems so that you can take any necessary corrective action to keep your service on track. That's your next step as a manager. Let's move on to Section IV, "Controlling."

IV

CONTROLLING

In previous sections we have discussed the managerial functions of planning, organizing, and directing. Under perfect conditions your job would be complete at this point. Unfortunately conditions in the real world are never perfect. For this reason you must ensure that you receive accurate information that reveals deviations from your expected results. Only in this way can you determine where the variances lie and implement the changes necessary to yield desired results.

What elements of your service require control? You should design control points in two key areas: performance (or quality) and finances. In Chapter 9, "Quality Control," we'll review techniques used to ensure that performance meets standards. In Chapter 10, "Controlling Your Finances," we'll review financial control.

Quality control

9

Control is crucial to the EMS concept. If we can't ensure that patients in fact receive high-quality emergency care from the street to the intensive care unit, then we're not doing our jobs.
—EMS PHYSICIAN

183

At this point you should be gaining confidence in your EMS management skills. After all, you know the fundamentals of planning, organizing, and directing. In this chapter you'll learn the next step in your management function—ensuring that your service and personnel actually achieve your objectives.

When you evaluate performance in EMS, you must do it on three levels. You must ensure that:

1. Personnel adequately perform those tasks described in the job descriptions developed in Chapter 3 through performance appraisal;
2. Your service meets the objectives that you developed for it in Chapter 2; and
3. Your service fulfills its obligations to the rest of the EMS system, specifically in the area of medical performance.

Ensuring performance through appraisal

Your personnel are the most important element in competent EMS performance. If your personnel don't do their jobs, you're sunk. As an EMS manager, you must ensure that your personnel perform their jobs up to the standards that you have set for them.[1] If you find that they aren't, you must develop a plan of action for improvement of performance. This process is called *performance appraisal,* and it has five steps:

1. Establish duties, qualities, standards, and goals consistent with the results that you desire.
2. Observe employee performance and compare it to your established standards.
3. Determine causes for deviations from standard and develop corrective plans.
4. Discuss your appraisal of performance with the employee.
5. Coach your employee as necessary.

1. Establish duties, qualities, standards, and goals.

In Chapter 3 we discussed the process of establishing effective job descriptions. At that point you might have thought job descriptions were tedious and a waste of time. Detailed job descriptions, however, are the basis for performance appraisal. If you did your work in Chapter 3 and wrote effective job descriptions, you'll be way ahead of other EMS managers when it comes to performance appraisal. As we said in Chapter 3, you must organize job duties, personal qualities, and standards on which you and your employees agree. If you don't, your employees will never know what you expect of them. Don't limit your employees' input to agreeing passively to the duties, qualities, and standards that you propose. Encourage your employees to develop their own performance goals, provided their goals mesh with the goals of your service. Be sure that you and your employee agree on standards of performance for these goals.

2. Observe performance and compare it to standards.

Once you and your employee have agreed on duties, qualities, standards, and goals, the employee should understand the job and your expectations for results. You then perform the following steps:

OBSERVE performance and measure it against the established standards. How do you observe performance? The most obvious way is to place yourself squarely within the employee's work area and observe (and listen). For EMS managers who provide direct patient care, this is relatively easy. You observe your personnel when you are working with them. Other EMS managers, however, may become tied to their desks. No matter how heavy your paper work burden, you must observe your employee's performance firsthand.

Direct observation isn't the only way to collect information. Use records whenever appropriate, such as patient charts or ambulance run forms, which demonstrate the amount and quality of work. You might review time cards for indications of dependability, absenteeism, and tardiness. You also might want to perform the employee's duties occasionally. If you can prepare the ambulance for the next run in 10 minutes while it takes Sam an hour, for example, you need to review Sam's performance.

DOCUMENT your observations. A pocket notebook comes in handy for this. Brief notes including dates and times are sufficient so long as you put your observations in writing. It's important to be as objective as possible when appraising performance. Don't rely on opinions when you have access to facts.

INFORM your employees of your findings. If your observations are positive, you have an opportunity to reinforce the behavior. If your observations are negative, you can show the employee what is wrong and explain how to correct it. In either event provide each employee with ongoing feedback concerning the quality of job performance. This way the actual appraisal interview will not come as a surprise, because it will merely summarize the message that the employee has been hearing from you.

COMPARE the observed performance to the standards as they appear in the job description. When you evaluate performance, you need only three rating levels:

1. Does not consistently meet standards.
2. Consistently meets standards.
3. Exceeds standards—innovative procedures or unusual effort has led to outstanding accomplishment.

Level 3 recognizes exceptional performance. In general the rating scale will focus on levels 1 and 2.

As you compare actual performance with standards, compile a list of all duties at or above standard and those duties below standard. Determine the three most critical duties from each category.

3. Determine causes for deviations from standards and develop corrective plans.

Your comparisons between standards and observed performance have resulted in a list of three critical job deficiencies. Your next step is to determine the causes for each deficiency. As managers, we often jump to the erroneous conclusion that job deficiencies are caused by a lack of interest on the employee's part or sheer laziness. You must avoid this type of shallow reasoning in favor of a lengthier but more accurate approach.[2] By asking

CONTROLLING yourself a series of questions about each deficiency you can zero in on exactly where the cause lies.

First consider the importance of the deficiency. Ask yourself, "What would happen if I left it alone?" If the answer is "nothing," then don't worry about it any further; it's not worth spending your valuable time trying to correct.

Assuming the deficiency is important, ask yourself a second set of questions: "Is a skill deficiency involved? Could the employee perform the duty properly if life depended on it?" Depending on your answers, you should continue your line of questions in one of two directions:

1. If the employee couldn't perform the duty properly even if life depended on it, it's a skill deficiency. Ask yourself the following questions:
   a. "Did the employee perform the duty properly in the past?" If the employee never knew how to perform the duty, arrange a training program.
   b. If the employee once knew how to perform the job properly but has forgotten, "Does the person perform the job often?" If the answer is no, you probably need to arrange for skill maintenance by providing a regular schedule of practice. If the answer is yes, you need to give the employee feedback on performance so that the person can improve it.
   c. "Is there a simple solution, such as providing job aids or storing needed information?" Written instructions or checklists, for example, can eliminate the need for the employee to remember all important details.
   d. "Does the employee have the physical and mental potential to perform as desired? Is the employee overqualified for the job?" If you answer either no to the first question or yes to the second question, you may have to consider transfer or termination.
2. If the employee could perform the duty properly if life depended on it, the problem is not a skill deficiency and the solution is not skill modification. Rather you must modify the conditions associated with performance. Ask yourself the following questions:
   a. "Is desired performance punishing?" If, for example, an EMT's positive performance is greeted with pressure from peers to slow down, the consequences

of proper performance are not reinforcing. You must modify the consequences so as to remove the punishment.

   b. "Is nonperformance rewarding?" If so, you should redesign the consequences so that proper performance is reinforced.

   c. "Does proper performance really matter to the employee?" If not, again you must design positive consequences.

   d. "Are there obstacles to performing?" Perhaps the standards that you have established are not clear enough for the employee, or the employee does not have the proper tools to do the job. Do whatever you must to remove these obstacles.

Once you have determined the cause of the deficiency and the likely cure, compare the size of the remedy with the size of the deficiency. If the solutions are inappropriate, impossible to implement, or beyond your resources, consider scaling down the solutions to yield the most result for the least cost or effort.

Remember that a single deficiency may have more than one cause; in that case, you may need to develop more than one corrective plan. Stay flexible as you go through this process, and remember that not all deficiencies are caused by the employee. You or the organization may be at fault. We've displayed this logical approach to determining the causes of employee deficiencies in Figure 9–1.

4. Discuss your appraisal of performance with the employee.

Most discussions of performance appraisal concentrate on the appraisal interview.[3,4,5] Although you should carefully plan for the interview, you should remember that frequent feedback to the employee during your observations provides a continuous appraisal process throughout the year. As such, if the specifics of your appraisal come as a surprise to the employee, you have failed to provide sufficient feedback on an ongoing basis.

The interview should focus on the critical job duties and standards that you selected when you compared actual performance to standards. In the interview you should

   1. Anticipate how the employee will react before you schedule the interview so that you aren't taken by surprise.

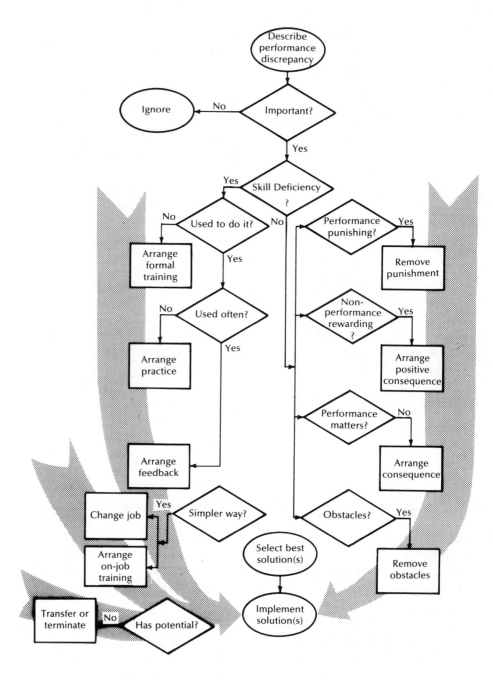

FIGURE 9-1.   Performance Analysis Grid

Reprinted with permission from R.F. Mager and P. Pipe, *Analyzing Performance Problems* (Belmont CA: Pitman Learning, Inc., 1970).

2. Provide the employee with advance notice of the inter-
    view.

3. Hold the interview in a private room. Allow sufficient
    time and give the interview your undivided attention.

4. Start the interview on a positive note by describing a job
    duty that meets or exceeds the standard. As you move on
    to duties that do not meet standards, sandwich them in
    between duties that do meet standards. Provide factual
    observations to support your evaluation.

5. Encourage the employee to talk. The person may reveal
    significant obstacles that preclude optimal perfor-
    mance. Ask directed questions when you need specific
    information, such as, "What do you think we should do
    about the increase in patient complaints?" Ask open-
    ended questions when you wish to encourage the em-
    ployee to open up, such as "Tell me about some of the
    frustrating problems that you have encountered." Your
    questions should encourage the employee to identify the
    causes and solutions for job deficiencies. An employee is
    far more likely to work toward solving the problem
    when he or she has identified it.

6. Maintain your flexibility during the interview. We all
    make mistakes, and if an employee points out an error in
    your appraisal, be willing to change your rating.

7. Pass on any secondhand compliments that you have
    heard. These act as particularly effective motivators.

8. Summarize the key points of the interview before clos-
    ing. Repeat all of the employee's positive points while
    highlighting those areas where the employee will work
    toward improvement.

9. If you promised to look into something during the inter-
    view, be sure to follow up on it and inform the employee
    of the result.

Remember: The emphasis of the appraisal interview should
be on performance, not on personality. If you follow our guidelines, the performance appraisal process should be a positive experience for both you and your staff, resulting in improved levels
of performance and increased morale.

How often should you perform a formal appraisal interview? If performed too frequently, the interview tends to em-

phasize day-to-day details at the expense of the bigger picture. If you delay too much between interviews, you lose both the opportunity to provide powerful motivation from recognition and the ability to improve a serious job deficiency. As a rough guide, you should consider holding an appraisal interview once every 6 to 12 months.

5. Coach the employee.

Managerial coaching consists of any activity in which the manager assists the employee to improve performance. Coaching is critical in effective performance appraisal; improvement in employee performance can take place only when you make a solid commitment to assist the employee in a meaningful way.

What avenues are open to you under the heading of coaching? Figure 9–1 can help point you in the right direction. Depending on your determination of the causes and solutions for job deficiencies, you might consider arranging formal training, developing opportunities for periodic maintenance, or providing meaningful feedback.

Before moving on to the next area of quality control, review Table 9–1, which summarizes the key points of the performance appraisal process. By applying these points to your service, you can effectively control the personnel resources available to you.

Ensuring your service meets its objectives

It's possible for your personnel to perform well, but your service to fail to meet its objectives. Chapter 2 provided you with the techniques for planning for your service. Those techniques will also provide you with the performance control that you need.

If you followed the guidelines presented in Chapter 2, you selected all or part of four systems for your service's planning. Here's how you use each of those plans for control.

Management by objectives

The performance standard in management by objectives (MBO) is the yearly objective. If your service is performing adequately, it will achieve its objectives. Missed objectives mean that your ser-

TABLE 9-1. Key Points of Performance Appraisal

Before the interview:

1. Review job duties, personal qualities, goals, and standards
2. Observe employee performance as carefully as possible.
3. Single out key strengths and weaknesses in performance.
4. Analyze possible causes of deviation from standard and develop a corrective plan.
5. Anticipate the employee's reaction to the interview.

At the interview:

1. Arrange for an undisturbed environment.
2. Open the interview on a positive note.
3. Sandwich negative points between positive ones.
4. Support your evaluation with hard data.
5. Use active listening techniques to encourage the employee to develop solutions first.
6. Summarize the interview.

After the interview:

1. Follow up on questions raised during the interview.
2. Use coaching techniques as indicated.

vice's performance is substandard. When your service misses an objective, ask yourself the following:

- Was the objective truly attainable?
- Were we organized adequately to achieve the objective?
- Did key administrative personnel reflect the objective in their monthly commitments?
- Did certain key administrative personnel fail to meet their commitments?
- Is the objective still worth pursuing?
- If so, how are we going to approach the objective so that this time we'll achieve it?

Suppose, for example, that one of your service's yearly commitments was to rewrite your disaster plan. The time frame was generous to achieve this objective. Your emergency department medical director was in charge of the project. Although he listed the disaster plan on his monthly commitments, he frequently stated his results as "in progress." You review the performance

193

with him and find that he didn't break the task down into doable pieces. He doesn't use a to-do list. His life goals and priorities are fouled up. You decide to have him read the first chapter of this book. You'll monitor his daily to-do lists and no longer allow him to put "in progress" as a result on his monthly commitments. By breaking the task into small pieces and completing them, he is able to complete the project.

Priority planning

The performance standard in priority planning (PP) is the minimal acceptable performance. Your priority planning profile will indicate when key elements of your service are substandard. Your service frequently will have a few substandard key elements. When many, or all, key elements are substandard, however, your service's performance is likely to be poor. When this happens, ask yourself the following:

- Have I set my minimal acceptable performance too high, or are we really doing a poor job?
- If we are doing a poor job, is there any pattern to my low rated key elements? Do they all deal with one area?
- When I evaluate the breakdown list of low-rated key elements, do certain poorly performed areas appear for several key elements?

Suppose, for example, that you direct a busy ambulance service and routinely delegate many tasks to your two assistant directors. When you review your priority profile, you find that several areas are below your minimal acceptable performance. The consistent pattern among all those areas is that they have been delegated to one of your two assistant directors. You review performance with that director and find that he has been ineffective due to serious family problems. You suggest that he take a leave of absence and he agrees. You call together a meeting of your key people and redelegate responsibility and authority. Service performance improves.

Managing for motivation

The performance standard in managing for motivation (MFM) consists of the scores on EMS attitude profiles. A score less than five on the profile means a negative attitude in an area that may have an impact on job satisfaction and motivation. When your profile scores are low, you must ask yourself the following:

- Is this poor motivation having an impact on the performance of my service?
- Is the poor motivation isolated to certain groups or individuals?
- Can I take steps to improve the problem?
- Are these steps likely to produce a positive result?

Suppose, for example, that you run a service that employs physicians, nurses, secretaries, and EMTs. You review the motivation profile and find that your employees' ratings of policies have slipped to a low level. You reanalyze your data and find that while the ratings of the physicians, nurses, and secretaries are holding steady, the EMTs' ratings have dropped significantly. You discuss the problem with your EMT supervisor and find that he feels that his staff's performance is also slipping. You discuss the matter with the EMTs, who state that the new overtime schedule policy is causing them serious problems. You discuss the issue with the supervisor, who then negotiates a new policy with his personnel. Performance returns to satisfactory levels.

Project evaluation and review technique

The performance standard in project evaluation and review technique (PERT) is the PERT chart on which you've listed the activities and events necessary to complete a major project. On the chart you've placed estimated times for completing each activity. When your service falls behind in meeting these time estimates, you may have performance problems. In such cases you must ask yourself the following:

- Were the time estimates reasonable?
- If the estimates are reasonable, which activities are falling behind schedule?
- Who is responsible for those activities and why are they having problems?
- Should you redesign those activities, turn them over to someone else, or provide more resources to complete them?

195

- Is it still reasonable to expect task completion?
- If so, by what date?

Suppose, for example, that you run a small ambulance service. Your board decided to upgrade your service from the basic to advanced level. Realizing that this involved a tremendous number of small tasks, you made a PERT chart and assigned different activities to members of your service. Halfway through the project you find that development of the new protocols is way behind schedule. This is important to you because writing the protocols falls on the critical path; a delay in the protocols will delay the whole project. You review the initial time estimates and realize that although they may have been realistic, you delegated the task to your most inexperienced person. As a result that person is overwhelmed. While you don't want to practice reverse delegation, you realize that you must speed up this activity. So you schedule more time with this person. You provide information on work planning from Chapter 1. You also inform your board that the upgrading will be completed slightly behind schedule and provide a revised target date. Your intervention works and you meet that new date.

The four examples demonstrate how you can apply planning techniques to ensuring that your service's performance meets expectations. Even if your personnel are performing adequately and your service is reaching its objectives, you may still have problems. That's because emergency medical services fit together to form a system. The system must provide adequate emergency health care from the street to the intensive care unit. As an EMS manager, you must ensure that your service fulfills its role in the system and that the system effectively discharges its responsibility to the public.

Ensuring your service fulfills its role

The provision of emergency medical care from the field to the intensive care units requires that different emergency medical services work cooperatively. As an EMS manager, you must ensure that the care provided meets acceptable medical standards. In EMS, this is called *medical control*. Here's what should happen: An EMT responds to an ill or injured patient and provides basic life support. When advanced life support skills are needed, the EMT performs them in accordance with training, current protocols, or instructions from the base station physician. On arrival at the hospital the emergency department physician provides competent emergency care. If necessary the patient is transferred to the inpatient service of the hospital.

Defining medical standards

As we've said, effective job descriptions provide standards for work performance. In the case of the EMT in the preceding example, one job standard might read, "Provides advanced life support care in accordance with good medical standards." In medical control, this statement is not adequate to ensure quality care. As a manager, you must not only ensure that the employee meets the standard to provide "care in accordance with good medical standards" but also define the good medical standards that the employee is to follow. When you define those standards, realize that

Medical care standards should be as precise as possible.

In EMS, small deviations from proper procedure can have disastrous consequences. The best way to define performance standards for prehospital care is to write protocols that carefully describe how the EMT is to perform in a given situation. An example of a protocol written for the management of seizures appears on the following page.

This protocol describes those advanced life support steps that a cardiac technician or paramedic should take in managing a patient who is actively seizing. (This particular protocol assumes that the cardiac technician or paramedic has already applied the required basic skills. In addition, it assumes that all patients weigh 70 kilograms. The protocol includes a drug dosage table for adjusting dosages for patients who weigh more or less than 70 kilograms.) Note that this protocol clearly describes what the cardiac technician or paramedic is to do in a particular medical situation. It provides for certain steps to be taken in all cases and other steps to be tailored to the needs of individual patients after the cardiac technician or paramedic has contacted the base hospital. This protocol avoids long discussions of the pathophysiology of seizures, controversies in treatment, or reasons why these particular steps were chosen. Effective protocols like this one are clear and to the point.

We asked the head nurse in a suburban emergency depart-

Protocol: Seizures

In managing patients who are actively seizing, the cardiac technician or paramedic will:

1. Administer oxygen through an established airway.

2. Start a dextrose 5 percent water intravenous infusion to keep the vein open.

3. Draw an appropriate blood tube for blood sugar determination.

4. Administer Thiamine 100 mg intravenously.

5. Administer dextrose 25 gm (50 cc of a 50 percent solution) intravenously.

6. Contact medical control for implementation of the following options.:

OPTION A: Diazepam 5–10 mg intravenously. (The rate is not to exceed 5 mg/min.) If the seizure has not stopped, the initial dose may be repeated.

OPTION B: Naloxone 0.8 mg intravenously if the possibility of drug ingestion exists.

ment for a copy of the protocols that directed the performance of prehospital personnel in her area. She handed us an old notebook. "Here they are," she said. "Nobody uses them any more; they're out-of-date." This is a common problem in EMS. Protocols, if not updated regularly, become useless.

Figure 9–2 demonstrates the natural history of protocols. Here's what happens: Members of an EMS system will decide that protocols need to be established. They will form a committee and work hard to write the protocols that describe the most effective medical treatment available at that time. After several months of labor they may produce a set of protocols on which everyone can agree. At that point medical care becomes fixed at a particular level. Because medical knowledge is always increasing, it isn't long before a gap appears between current medical knowledge and the medical treatment described in the protocols. As a result the protocols will be partially out-of-date within six

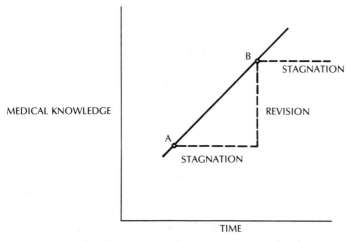

The solid line represents the level of emergency medical knowledge.
The dotted line represents how EMS protocols reflect current knowledge.
Point A is the point where the protocols are written.
Point B is the point where the protocols are revised.

FIGURE 9–2. Natural History of EMS Protocols

months. The committee members are generally tired of working
on the protocols at that time and have no desire to rewrite them.
Care becomes fixed at the level of the initial writing of the protocols because no one has the energy to keep them up-to-date.
When the gap between current medical knowledge and the pre-
scribed medical treatment becomes great enough, EMS personnel will stop using the protocols and the medical control system
begins to unravel.

We spoke with a state EMS director whose state had developed a series of protocols under federal grants several years
previously. "I know that they're out-of-date," he said. "But I no
longer have the resources to undertake the job of rewriting
them." His state's protocols were no longer used in the routine
care of patients.

As an EMS manager, when you are presented with the pros-
pect of your system's developing prehospital protocols, consider
how you plan to keep them up-to-date. To keep your protocols up-
to-date, you must do two things:

1. You must have a core of committed EMS personnel who
    have the authority to prepare protocols for your region.
    These must be people who have the authority to agree on
    issues and have the ability to negotiate differences

cooperatively. Such a committee is not the place for physicians or EMTs who are "always right" or at the other extreme, indecisive. This core of people must be up-to-date and well-read in the EMS literature. Their decisions in committee meetings will affect hundreds of people in the streets.

2. You must have a system that can readily update the current protocols to reflect changes made by the committee. The simplest way is with a word-processing system. You can set up a system on the most modest microcomputer. Once the initial protocols have been typed into the word processor, periodic revision is easy. A committee can meet regularly, decide on the necessary changes, and generate a new set of updated protocols without difficulty. Once you have implemented a system that enables rapid revision of protocols, however, you may develop a problem. Prehospital personnel must be comfortable with your protocols. If the protocols change too often, your personnel will lose track of what the current protocol is. In revising your protocols you must select a time frame that keeps them up-to-date without making too many unnecessary changes. Try six months as an initial time frame for revisions.

Ensuring personnel follow medical standards

Defining medical standards is not enough to ensure effective medical control. You must also ensure that your personnel follow those standards. In the first part of this chapter we discussed dealing with performance that does not meet appropriate job standards. Much of that discussion applies to medical control. However, you must recognize a few other special considerations.

Training vs. education

In Chapter 3 we discussed the difference between education and training. This difference will affect your approach to medical control. Because a trained person will respond to an emergency by doing what has been taught, your approach to medical control must guarantee that the person has been taught the proper action and carries it out. On the other hand, because an educated person responds to an emergency by drawing on a broad base of knowledge and reaching a decision regarding action, you must ensure that the education has provided an adequate base of knowledge and that the reasoning is sound.

Training programs must include the medical standards that you have selected. If you hire a new EMT from another area, don't assume that the person knows the specifics of your protocols. To exert competent medical control, you must train the EMT in those protocols.

In ensuring medical control over educated personnel like EMS physicians, you will need to use other tools to ensure that the physician's education has been adequate to reach competent EMS decisions. Many of us remember that when esophageal-obturator airways were first used, physicians would pull them out saying, "What's this damn thing?" *A medical degree is no assurance of competence in EMS.*

One way to ensure the quality of physician training is to extend the standard physician credentialing process to emergency medicine. When physicians join hospital medical staffs, they must request privileges. Medical staff credentialing committees have generally not assessed EMS skills. This oversight means that base-station instructions to prehospital personnel may not reflect current medical standards. If this is a problem in your system, push for more stringent credentialing.

Retrospective control mechanisms

Adopting standardized protocols and ensuring that your personnel are competently trained are prospective methods of medical control in that you complete these steps before an emergency occurs. They improve the likelihood that your personnel will provide competent emergency medical care. In addition to these prospective techniques you need retrospective controls.

Retrospective controls examine care after it has been delivered to assure that it is in accordance with accepted standards. There are three approaches to retrospective control that you will use: outcome audits, decision-making analysis, and protocol-exception review.

OUTCOME AUDITS. Outcome audits are the most commonly employed method of retrospective medical control. Outcome audits answer questions about the quality of care delivered

201

by your system and point out ways in which care might be improved. For example, you might ask whether cardiac arrest patients had a better survival rate in your region if they were transported by an advanced-life-support unit as opposed to a basic unit. There are four basic steps in an outcome audit.

1. **Clearly state the question you are trying to answer.** "We need to do an audit." How often have you heard that in EMS? If your goal in auditing cases is merely to *do* an audit, you'll probably select the easiest topic to study and learn little of value. The real purpose of an audit is to answer a specific, important question. State that question as clearly as possible; for example, "Do patients treated prophylactically with lidocaine have better survival from myocardial infarctions?"

2. **Select a study population and methods.** Once you've determined the question that you want to answer, you must select your study population. For example, if you're studying systemwide ambulance response time, whom are you going to examine? You might examine all calls over a two-day period, for example, or every third call over a four-day period, or all calls every other day over a six-day period, or 50 randomly selected calls over a one-month period. Your population selection must be a compromise between accuracy and practicality. You'll want to select the most representative group that will provide you with the answer to the question that you've raised. However, you must keep that group small enough that you can perform the study.

   After you've determined your population, you must select the methods that you're going to use. Will the study be prospective (examining calls in the future) or retrospective (looking back at previous calls)? Will you use information that you're already gathering, or will you have to gather a new set of information? How will you gather the data? How will you store it?

3. **Collect and analyze data.** Next you must collect the data that you need in the fashion determined in the previous section. Many people manipulate data in order to prove the point that they want to make. Avoid that by being as objective as possible. Whenever you can, analyze your

results to determine if they are statistically significant. Computers are often helpful in handling audit data and determining statistical significance.

4. **Make recommendations.** If your audit proved that a particular type of therapy or procedure had a positive impact on patient outcome, translate that observation into management recommendations for your system. If you found that triage nurses significantly reduced patient waiting time in emergency departments, for example, recommend a full-scale evaluation of their expanded use.

These are the four basic steps in conducting outcome audits. For further information in conducting audits, consult a text that discusses this subject in depth.[6]

DECISION–MAKING ANALYSIS. Because educated personnel call on their broad base of knowledge and decide the best approach to an emergency, you must evaluate that decision-making process to see if errors are being made. To do this, review cases in depth and in their proper time sequence. In an emergency, decisions made out of order or too late can have serious consequences. The format shown in the exhibit on the following page provides an effective means of displaying cases for a review of decision making.

This review provides a means of evaluating the order and timing of the steps taken in the care of this case. This provides you with an orderly way to determine errors in the decision making of the practitioner who directed the case.

PROTOCOL–EXCEPTION REVIEW. An effective means of evaluating cases where trained personnel have delivered care is through a protocol-exception review. If you have defined medical performance standards carefully, you can effectively review performance by examining those cases where your trained personnel provided care that deviated from standard. In some cases, deviation may be justified. In other cases, deviation from performance standard may highlight fundamental problems with performance. This technique represents an example of management by exception in medical control. We'll discuss the concept of management by exception further in Chapter 10.

CASE 26:   82-year-old female   Date: January 13, 1983

HISTORY: · 82-year-old female was having increased chest pain this afternoon and ap-
                  parently passed out for a few seconds. Patient's son caught her and kept her
                  from falling down. He brought her inside and laid her on the couch. Patient
                  vomited x 1. History of heart problem, pacemaker implant 9/10/82. No known
                  allergies. Medications: Nitro, Digoxin, Verapamil, and Librium.

PREHOSPITAL: Ambulance at the scene at 2:50 p.m.

      minutes
         0   conscious, alert, and oriented
                  diaphoretic
                  shortness of breath
                  chief complaint—chest pain
                  oxygen administered 2L/M via nasal cannula
         5   B/P—140/78; P—88 irregular; R—24
                  pupils equal and reactive
                  skin wet and warm
         6   Nitro given SL
        11   Nitro given SL
        12   I.v. D5W started with 18 ga. in right forearm TKO
                  EKG junctional rhythm with occasional return to pacemaker rhythm
                  oxygen at 4 L/M
                  Medical Control contacted
        20   M.S. 2.5 mg adminstered i.v.
                  marked ectopic activity (multifocal PVCs)
        22   B/P—108 by palpation
                  P—90 irregular; R—36 wheezes
                  pupils equal and reactive—sluggish
                  skin wet and warm
        25   Lidocaine 35 mg administered i.v.
                  most PVCs abolished
                  chest pain relieved but some discomfort still noted
                  dyspnea increased
                  level of consciousness diminished
                  not responsive to verbal & touch stimuli
                  oxygen 8 L/M via face mask
                  Medical Control contacted
        39   M.S. 2.5 mg administered i.v.
        40   40-mg Lasix administered
                  transported in Fowlers position
        41   B/P—80 palpation
                  P—92 irregular; R—36 wheezes
                  pupils NRL
                  skin wet and warm
                  B/P—30 by palpation
                  level of consciousness down

43 0.8-mg Narcan i.v. push
no change in blood pressure
no change in level of consciousness
radial pulse weak—barely palpated
respiratory arrest
patient placed in supine position
intubated with 6.5-ET tube
BV oxygen 10 L/M
bagged 25 per minute

EMERGENCY ROOM ARRIVAL—3:45 p.m.

minutes
0 unconscious
diaphoretic
neck veins distended on exam
responsive to pain
not responsive to questions
5 ABGs drawn
P—80
R—began breathing on her own sporadically
bagged almost continuously
12 P—98 doppler
18 1-amp Bicarb given
25 1-amp Bicarb given
blood drawn for CBC, BUN, glucose, lytes and cardiac enzymes
EKG done
chest x-ray done
32 B/P—102/58; P—84; R—40
very diaphoretic
38 Lasix 40 mg given i.v.
40 Aminophyllin drip 0.5 mg/kg/ml
41 ABGs drawn
45 B/P—70/40
bagged
47 Aminophyllin drip 0.5 mg/kg/ml
i.v. team
50 125-mg Bolus
54 1-amp Bicarb given
Aminophyllin stopped—saline flush
60 admitted to ICU
diaphoretic
unresponsive
intubated—breathing assisted

ASSESSMENT: CHF, probably secondary to myocardial infarction, possibility of pulmonary embolus

Summary

As an EMS manager, you must ensure that the tasks that you have carefully planned and organized actually occur. First, you must measure your staff's work against performance standards. Second, you must determine whether your service is meeting the objectives that you developed in Chapter 2. Third, you must ensure that your service is fulfilling its role in delivering quality medical care within the EMS system. Whenever you spot deviations from adequate performance, you must take steps to correct them.

Ensuring adequate performance is a major step in effective EMS management. To be successful, you also need to control another major area: finances. High-quality emergency medical care is impossible unless you have the money to pay for it. In the next chapter we'll discuss how to collect the money that you need to support your service.

10

Controlling your finances

My biggest problem is collections. In a sense, collections are the most important problem in EMS. After all, if you can't get the money to pay for your services, everything else becomes meaningless.
—*EMT, OWNER AND MANAGER OF AN AMBULANCE SERVICE*

The EMS manager in the above quote puts the importance of financial control in its proper perspective: "... if you can't get the money to pay for your services, everything else becomes meaningless." In the previous nine chapters you learned much of what you need to be a successful EMS manager. No matter how well you've learned those lessons, if you don't control your finances, you'll fail in EMS management.

In Chapter 4 you learned how to organize your service's finances. If you apply those principles to your service, you've done half your job as a financial manager. This chapter teaches you the other half of that job. You must determine whether the projections of volume that you made have actually occurred. You must ensure that your actual expenses don't exceed expectations. You must be certain that the revenues that you projected actually were generated and collected. In the real world of EMS management financial problems develop no matter how well you applied the lessons of Chapter 4. Our job is to examine how you are going to find out where your financial problems are and what you're going to do about them.

Designing a format for financial control

Your first step in developing a system of financial control is to design a format for comparing your service's actual performance to the forecasts that you developed in Chapter 4. You must design a format that will help you in investigating differences between actual and expected financial performance. Your format should present your actual and expected performances side by side to underscore the comparison. A third column of numbers—the variance or difference between actual and expected—emphasizes the comparison even further. Table 10–1 displays part of an ambulance service financial performance report.

As you can see, Table 10–1 consists of the same three segments that you developed forecasts for in Chapter 4: volume of service, expenses, and revenues. In addition, expenses are further subdivided into salaries, supplies, and depreciation. These in turn are subdivided even further.

"Wait a minute," you might be thinking. "How many items

TABLE 10–1. Ambulance Service Financial Performance Report

	CURRENT MONTH			YEAR TO DATE		
	ACTUAL	BUDGET	VARIANCE	ACTUAL	BUDGET	VARIANCE
Volume of service						
Ambulance runs						
Expenses						
Salaries:						
EMTs (advanced)						
EMTs (basic)						
Attendants						
Clerical						
Administrative						
Total salaries						
Supplies						
Drugs						
IVs						
Medical/surgical						
Medical gasses						
Nonchargeable						
Total supplies						
Depreciation						
Vehicles						
Equipment						
Buildings						
Other						
Total depreciation						
Miscellaneous						
expenses						
Total expenses						
Revenues						
Patient charges						
Less:						
(Bad debts)						
(Third party						
allowances)						
Net revenues						

am I going to keep track of? If I start subdividing supplies, for example, I could make a list that goes on for pages?" You raise an important point. On the one hand the more subdivisions you have, the more involved and time-consuming your system of financial control becomes. On the other hand the more subdivisions you can add to your format, the easier it will be to track down problems. It's easier to determine what's going on, for example, if you specifically know that your drug expenses are higher than expected rather than if you generally know that your total supply expenses are higher than expected. No single format is "best" for your financial performance report. Much depends on the nature of your own service. However, the principle that you should follow is this:

Make your format as in-depth as you possibly can, considering the data-processing limitations of your service.

From this it should be clear that if you can computerize the processing of information for your report, you'll be better off than if you try to do it by hand. We'll talk more about computer systems later in this chapter.

Accurately reporting management data

Once you've designed your format, you need to develop a system to collect reliable information for it. To do this, you need to develop reporting mechanisms that will provide you with adequate information of volume, expenses, and revenues.

VOLUME. Most services rely on a run report form or a log to keep track of the volume of service. These systems usually work well unless they are overwhelmed by high volumes, in which case a computerized report form is necessary.

EXPENSES. When collecting information about expenses, you must determine whether you are going to gather information on a cash or an accrual basis. Under a cash basis you generate an expense whenever you write a check. You can design a cash system fairly easily. You simply keep a monthly record of each category of expense listed on your financial performance report, adding an entry to the appropriate category whenever a check is written. At the end of each month you add up each category and enter the total on your financial performance report.

Generating your expenses on an accrual basis is more time-consuming but more accurate. Under an accrual system you generate an expense when you use a service rather than when you pay for it. As an example, suppose that you pay your personnel every two weeks and the last day of the month is in the middle of the pay period. Under an accrual system you would include one week's worth of salaries on the financial performance report for the month just ended, even though your employees have not yet been paid for that week. As a result, by using an accrual method your report accurately reflects the costs of services that you have used during the month, whether you have paid for them yet or not.

If you decide to use an accrual system, you will need to develop a system to determine when expenses are generated. This will be more complicated than just keeping track of your checks. Often you can use a computer to track your ongoing expenses.

In EMS, managers use both accrual and cash systems for their financial performance reports. Either system is acceptable. Which you use will depend on the accuracy you require and the data-processing and clerical services at your disposal.

REVENUES. To collect information about revenues, you need to develop a reporting system for charges. The best way to do this is to collect the information at the time of service. Your staff plays a major role in this type of system because they will actually be filling out a charge ticket. Your ticket should be simple, while still gathering all necessary information. Depending on the nature of your service, this information might include medications, IVs, other supplies, room fees, professional fees, mileage, and time charges.

Utilizing variance analysis

At this point you should understand how to design a financial performance report that fits your service's needs and how to collect accurate information for that report. The next step is to use the report to improve your financial control.

Your financial performance report may have dozens of items listed on it. How do you know which of those items deserve your attention? Remember the 80/20 rule from Chapter 1. Eighty percent of your financial problems will stem from 20 percent of the items on your report.

Because of random fluctuations (particularly over a short

period of time) you should not expect actual results to match your budget figures exactly in any single budget area. You certainly don't want to investigate each difference between actual and budget; you don't have enough time. You're only interested in the 20 percent that are causing problems. So you must develop ranges of acceptable variance, investigating only those situations that deviate from the acceptable range. In the case of total EMT salaries, if your monthly budget is $10,000, you might establish an acceptable range of $9,500 to $10,500. If you have computerized your budgeting process, you can design your financial performance report program to highlight those variances that exceed plus or minus $500. This illustrates the concept of management by exception, where you concentrate on the important deviations from budgeted expectations; you don't waste your valuable time on those parts of the report that reflect the smoothly running aspects of your service.[1]

When you identify significant variances, you'll probably find them in three major areas: Your actual volume of work or revenues will be lower than expected or your expenses will be higher than expected.

Lower than predicted volume of work

When we discussed the development of budget projections in Chapter 4, we emphasized the importance of conservative forecasts of volume of work. When your volume of work is significantly less than what you projected, you'll have problems because your revenues will also be significantly less than you expected. What are some of the causes of lower than expected volumes of work?

- **Inadequate data base for projections.** If you haven't kept adequate statistics in the past on utilization, your forecasted volume may be high.

- **Incorrect interpretation of data.** If you incorrectly drew the "best line" described in Chapter 4 to predict your future volume, your forecasted volume may be high.

- **Declining quality of service.** If the public perceives your service as lacking quality, your actual volume of service may decrease.

- **Increased rates.** As noted in Chapter 4 one of the risks of raising your rates is declining utilization.

- **Increased competition.** If another ambulance service opened in the area and you did not take its impact into account when you prepared your forecast, your actual volume of service may be lower than expected.

- **Unforeseen technical problems.** If you had mechanical difficulty with your ambulances or the road leading to your emergency department was under repair, you may have a less than expected volume of service.

- **Worsening economic times.** In bad economic times people often postpone health care. This may cause your volume of service to decrease.

- **Changing physician patterns.** A change in the number or type of physicians in your area may affect volume of service.

- **Changing accident or illness patterns.** There is often a year-to-year variation in the incidence of certain infectious diseases that may affect your volumes. In addition, changes in the public's enthusiasm for certain dangerous sports may affect your volume.

If your actual volume of service fails to meet your projections, look for some of the preceding factors in your service. If you identify one, take steps to correct it if possible.

Higher than predicted expenses

When you spot significantly higher expenses than you forecasted, you need to examine four possible causes: increased volume of service, decreased productivity, increased hourly salary expense, or increased unit supply costs.

- **Increased volume of service.** Remember our discussion of variable costs in Chapter 4. Many of your expenses are variable with respect to your volume of work. As such, when your ambulance service transports more patients, for example, you can expect your supply expense to increase. As long as your supply expense per transport does not increase, this should not cause any problems. Sometimes, however, EMS expenses increase faster than volume of service. If increased ambulance runs have forced you to pay more overtime, for example, your salary expense per run might increase. For this reason it's important that you don't assume that increased volume of service will explain all your increased expenses. When expenses exceed projections, even in the presence of increased volumes of service, you must investigate three other possible causes.

Controlling
your
finances

- **Decreased productivity.** In Chapter 3 you learned to evaluate an EMS unit of work (ambulance run or patient visit) and organize your personnel to produce the amount of work that you expect. Suppose, for example, that you direct an ambulance service and you determined through work measurement the amount of time required for an ambulance run. When you developed your budget, you forecasted your salary expense based on four EMT hours per run. If your actual number of EMT hours per run is six, you have a productivity problem. Productivity may be low because of poor job descriptions, low motivation, overstaffing, or equipment problems. Once you've identified the specific reasons for productivity problems in your service, you can take appropriate steps to correct them through reorganizing your service's work or intervening through the performance appraisal process.

- **Increased hourly salary expense.** It's possible that your service is meeting its productivity expectations and yet is experiencing higher than expected total salary costs. This can happen if you exceed your forecast for hourly wage rates in one or more categories. If you find your forecast for EMT wage per hour in the budget period is $7, for example, but your actual wage per hour is $9.50, you've identified one possible reason for your increased costs. In EMS, actual hourly wage rates exceed the budget because of extensive overtime, unanticipated upgrading of skills, unexpected raises in pay, effects of hiring higher skilled or experienced personnel, or lack of an adequate system of budgeting costs. If you applied the job-rating system outlined in Chapter 4, this last item will not be a problem for you. Once you identify why your unit salary costs are too high, you can take steps to correct them. If you found that you are paying too much overtime, for example, you could hire additional part-time personnel.

- **Increased unit supply costs.** In Chapter 4 we discussed unit costs. Applying the unit cost concept to your supply

215

expenses provides you with valuable information. Suppose, for example, that you direct an emergency department, and you forecast a total supply budget of $100,000 for 25,000 patient visits. Your budgeted unit supply cost would be $4. If you actually spend $150,000 for 30,000 visits, then your actual unit supply cost is $5. There could be several explanations for this increase in unit supply costs: (1) inflation might be exceeding your estimate; (2) your patient population could be changing in character, causing an increase in supply usage; (3) your purchasing practices may be ineffective, or (4) someone may be stealing from your inventory. If your actual unit supply cost exceeds your forecast, try to determine the exact cause and apply the appropriate corrective action.

Lower than predicted revenues

Revenues vary with volume. If your revenues are less than projected, but your revenue per unit of work is equal to what you projected, then you have a problem with volume, not revenues. If, however, your revenue per unit of work is less than projected, you have a revenue problem.

In Chapter 4 you learned that forecasting revenues can be extremely difficult because what you charge isn't necessarily what you'll be able to put in the bank. When your revenues are less than expected, and it's not solely a volume problem, then your service is either not billing for proper amounts or not collecting bills at the rate that you forecast.

- **Inadequate charging.** If you find that your charge per unit of service is less than expected, either you overestimated the true charge per unit of service (in which case you need to review the data base from which you made your projection), or your personnel aren't correctly filling in charge forms. If you find that your personnel are having difficulty with the charge forms, discuss the situation with them. Remember: You didn't enter EMS for the money and neither did your personnel. As a result, charging is probably a low-priority item for them. Make your charging system simple. Train your personnel carefully. If possible, study profiles of your individual personnel to see whose charges are low and target your training to those people. Make sure that your charge slips are actually sent to the people who do your billing. If you carefully monitor the charging process, you can find your problem.

- **Inadequate collections.** Correcting problems with collections can be more difficult than correcting charging problems. If you manage a hospital-based emergency medical service, you probably aren't concerned about collecting payment from your patients: Your hospital undoubtedly has a fully staffed credit and collections department, which handles all payment issues. If you manage a private ambulance service, on the other hand, cash flow is probably a daily concern.

When it comes to collections, you should consider two key goals. The first is to collect payment on your bills (receivables) as quickly as possible. This provides you with cash to meet your expenses. Early collection of your receivables also improves your position with regard to the time value of money: A patient bill collected today can be invested to yield a greater sum than the same bill collected next month. You should target a maximum number of days in receivables that you wish to carry. You calculate days in receivables by comparing your current outstanding receivables to the average revenue your service generates per day. Suppose that you have $100,000 in outstanding receivables. If your service generates $1,000 per day, your days in receivables equals:

$$\frac{\$100,000}{\$1,000/\text{day}} = 100 \text{ days}$$

Your first goal should be to minimize this figure. Specifying your goal in this manner will assist you later in determining if you have met your target.

The second goal concerns your service's relationship with the public. You should work as cooperatively as possible with patients in the receivables process so as to minimize antagonism with your community. If you practice a heavy-handed approach, you may find that patients refuse to use your service. All of your other efforts toward providing a high-quality service would then be wasted.

Once you have established your goals, consider how quickly you wish to follow up on outstanding patient accounts. Use your targeted number of days in receivables for guidance here. Clearly the fewer days you wish to carry in receivables, the quicker your follow-up must begin. Generally you will find yourself somewhat limited by insurance company practices. Given the wide variety of insurance policies that cover emergency services, it is difficult to know how much of a bill will remain the responsibility of the patient. You can usually expect to wait up to 60 days for insurance payments, which thus represents a minimum period before you can actually begin a follow-up.

Next consider the minimum balance that justifies a full-scale collection effort. Assuming that your service operates at a relatively busy pace, you will have a large number of open accounts, many of which are fairly small. Although you should send an initial statement to all patients, followed up by a reminder, it is questionable whether further efforts are justified for small balances. You must be the judge of what constitutes a small balance given the context of your own service.

For larger balances you should determine the methodology that you intend to employ with respect to follow-up efforts. Will you send letters or make phone calls? At what point will you hand accounts over to collection agencies or attorneys? Once you answer these questions, you can use work measurement techniques to determine how many people you'll need to handle your service's collection needs. When you hire employees for collection work, be sure that you choose assertive, extroverted individuals; after all, collection is no place for someone who is afraid of talking to people.

Computers are helpful in collection, because they can quickly sort data in a variety of ways. You gain an excellent means for directing your collection effort if you sort the data by age of account. Such aged-trial balances offer you immediate information on the age and extent of the receivables that you are carrying. You can also sort your receivables by head of household. This array provides a useful working tool for following up on collections.

Before beginning any collection efforts with a patient, you should determine insurance coverage. Insurance policies vary widely as far as their specific terms and conditions. Many require the patient to pay a deductible figure before the policy begins to pay. Often the patient must pay a certain percentage (called a *copayment*) as well, such as 20 percent of the total bill. Be sure that you understand exactly what the policy pays and what the patient is responsible for before contacting the patient.

Once you have identified the patient's portion of the bill, send a billing statement to the patient. Generally a second statement should be mailed before initiating any phone calls. If a phone call is necessary, remember the negotiating techniques described in Chapter 6. Use a cooperative approach, because this takes advantage of the typical situation, where a patient honestly wants to work with you. Emphasize to the patient that you will do whatever you reasonably can to help. Suggest possible arrangements for payments over time if the patient is financially strapped. Although you should ask for the full balance, recognize that you may have to settle for less. Seek input from the patient as far as the timing of payments, but try to maximize the amount that the patient pays each period. You should establish a minimum payment per period (our minimum is $20) and stick to it. Keep accurate records of the terms of these arrangements, as well as subsequent payments. Keep on top of the payment agreements you establish, and follow up promptly if defaults occur.

If a patient is unwilling to cooperate, will not make contact with you, or has a previous record of poor payments, consider referring the account to either a collection agency or an attorney. The courtroom approach is preferable if you know that the patient owns significant assets, because the court will likely order an award to you.

Your most direct control over collections is the aged-trial balance referred to earlier. This document, which is easily generated if your receivables are logged on a computer, tells you how many days of receivables you are carrying. You therefore have a quick and simple control point comparing actual days against the targeted number of days that you established as your goal.

You can generate other pieces of information to refine your control further. You can calculate the collection rate of any clerks to whom you have delegated the receivables work, comparing this rate against an established standard of performance. Likewise, you can calculate a targeted rate for any collection agency that you employ. If the actual rate falls significantly below a predetermined amount (15 percent, for example), it's an indication that the agency is not performing properly. Employing two agencies and comparing their collection records provides further insights on this. If the rate exceeds the predetermined target, you are probably forwarding to the agency accounts that you could have collected on your own. As a result you may have needlessly forfeited the commissions that the agency will collect.

Applying computers to control systems

We've frequently mentioned the value of applying computers to certain EMS management tasks, particularly in this chapter on financial control. Table 10–2 lists some of the computer applications in EMS. Because many of the financial control mechanisms in EMS are best performed by computer, you must understand how to use computer systems so that they provide you with the needed control.

In examining how computer systems have been applied in EMS, we've found that certain problems seem to recur continually. If you apply five basic principles, you can reduce these problems.

1. Avoid computer jargon whenever possible.

We spoke with the president of a large emergency medical corporation. His organization had lost over a quarter of a million dollars in a computer software venture. Discussing the reasons

TABLE 10–2. EMS Computer Applications

1. Sorting Data
   a. Generating performance reports (211)
   b. Listing open accounts receivable by age of account or head of household (218)
   c. Performing audits (203)
2. Routine Calculations
   a. Generating salary forecasts (100)
   b. Calculating variances (213)
3. Statistical Calculations
   a. Calculating linear regressions (97)
   b. Calculating statistical significance (203)
   c. Calculating staffing levels by patient volume analysis (80)
4. Modeling
   a. Examining effects of expansion of patient service area (98)
5. Word Processing
   a. Keeping protocols up-to-date (200)
   b. Maintaining job descriptions (75)

Note: Number in parenthesis is the number of the page where item is discussed in text.

for that loss, he said, "The guy we had in charge of the program was incompetent, but I was late in discovering that because he always spoke in computer jargon and I didn't understand what he was saying. The vice president, who managed our computer operations, acted like he knew what was going on, but he didn't know any more about it than I did."

Effective communication is essential to good management. Computer jargon short-circuits communication. While the jargon can save time when one computer person is talking to another, it intimidates noncomputer people. As a manager, make sure that you understand what your computer people are saying to you. Use your active listening techniques. Don't be afraid to ask a dumb question because you don't understand jargon. Often you will find that jargon can cover up sloppy thinking.

2. Don't computerize any task that doesn't need to be computerized.

We spoke with a member of a committee considering computerizing a local United Way. He said, "We're thinking about getting a computer. Other local areas use them. We have an executive and a secretary in the office now who do most of the work and they do a good job. I wonder whether a computer will improve upon that. Will it be cost-effective?" Computers are seductive. Without experience in computers, it's easy for a manager to think that computers are going to solve every problem. In fact computers rarely solve problems; they just substitute one set of problems for another. You must carefully select those tasks that you are going to computerize. Ask yourself, "Is that task being performed adequately without computers?" If it is, don't computerize it. Ignore the claims of computer people who say that they can improve your performance on that task. You don't need them.

3. If you computerize an important task, make sure that you have a back-up system.

In our region we decided to computerize our prehospital protocols with a microcomputer. Shortly after we implemented this system, the computer broke down for six weeks. Computers break down; you can count on it. If you are considering computerizing an important task, follow these suggestions:

- Never rely on a single computer that has no backup.
- If possible in a system, use several compatible small computers instead of one larger one. When one computer breaks down, your system can still function.
- Whenever possible, select computer components that are plugged-in rather than built-in. Computer systems with all the components built into a cabinet are good-looking, but when one component fails, the whole computer often doesn't work. With plugged-in components you can usually unplug the defective component and replace it. You don't lose the use of the computer.
- Never buy a computer that doesn't have reliable, easily available repair service.

4. Remember that software is more important than hardware.

We spoke with the head of a computer corporation that develops health-related computer systems. He said: "For the most part, software (computer programs) is more important than hardware (the machines themselves). You can always find several good computers that will solve a problem; the difficulty is to find good programs to run them." Good software in EMS is scarce. If you are installing a computer system, you will either have to write your own programs or adapt programs developed from other areas. Your use of computers will be limited by the lack of good software, not the inadequacy of hardware. Don't make your computer decisions based on hardware alone.

5. Don't computerize meaningless or redundant information.

We spoke with the president of a group of private ambulance services that had recently been computerized. He said: "Our biggest mistake in starting to use computers was to expect the computer to do everything. After each ambulance run, we'd spend about 10 minutes entering data into the computer. Much of that data was already being analyzed by the state, so we were just duplicating their work. We got so that we were entering so much information, we had little time to use the computer for more important things."

Computer people have a saying, "Garbage in, garbage out." You must ensure that you are entering only meaningful information into your computer and that your computer is providing you

with the information you need. If your computer buries you in irrelevant information, it will become more of a hindrance than a
help.

Summary

In this chapter you've learned how to ensure that the financial
forecasts that you made in Chapter 4 actually occur. By applying
the principles of variance analysis, you can identify where your
service is failing to meet your projections and what steps you can
take to correct that failure. Without the money to pay for it, no
EMS service can operate. By applying the guidelines for collections that you learned here, you can make sure that the money
you budgeted actually ends up in your service's bank account.

The computer age will bring new capabilities and challenges
to EMS management. Throughout this book you've learned about
numerous computer applications. Computers are extremely
helpful in controlling your finances, but you must be able to control the computer. The five principles that you learned here will
help you.

At this point in traditional management books you'd be finished with your training; you know how to plan, organize, direct,
and control. If you apply those techniques in EMS, your service
might thrive, but you might not. We started this book by saying
that your first job as an EMS manager is to manage yourself. To
manage yourself and your service requires that you survive as a
manager. Let's take steps to ensure your survival.

SURVIVING

In Chapter 11, "Managing Stress," we will help you assess the impact that stress is having on your health and your job performance, show you how your personality can influence the way that stress affects you, and provide you with techniques that can help you control stress before it kills you.

11

Managing stress

I would go to training classes and they would take my blood pressure and ask me if I knew it was high. I would pass off their comments. Then one day, I really looked at myself. I had hypertension, felt run down, and was overweight. I was working all the time, eating junk meals while I was on the run. I went to my doctor. He asked me a lot of questions: How many hours was I working? Was I happy? and so on. I began to realize the effect the stress of work was having on me. I enjoy my work and I want to do it well. But I enjoy my family, too. After that, I changed the way I did things. I decided to take time to stop and smell the roses.
—EMT, DIRECTOR OF AMBULANCE SERVICE

Stress. Instinctively you know what it is. As an EMS manager, stress is your constant companion. It causes the uneasy feeling in the pit of your stomach when you are racing to the scene of an automobile accident, the sweaty palms when you stand to make a presentation to the state EMS meeting, the pounding pulse when you sit down to terminate a problem employee.

We are living in what has been called the Age of Anxiety, and stress has become an inescapable fact of life for everyone. What makes it worse for you is that you are not just dealing with management problems, but are handling life-and-death situations. More than anything else, you must learn to understand and control stress if you are to be an effective manager—and survive.

What is stress?

Stress is defined as *a specific group of physical and emotional responses that occur in reaction to a variety of demands—positive and negative, physical and emotional.* This definition contains three points that are fundamental to your understanding of stress.

1. Stress is a specific group of physical and emotional responses.

Think back to the last time when you were undergoing a lot of stress. How did you feel? Chances are that you felt several of these symptoms:

- Your heart was pounding.
- Your pulse was racing.
- Your palms were sweaty.
- Your throat was dry.
- You had "butterflies" in your stomach.
- You were breathing faster.
- You were shaking inside.
- You felt tense and nervous.

Walter B. Cannon, a physiology professor at the Harvard Medical School, first described the physical effects of stress in the early 1900s.[1] He called it the *fight-or-flight response*. The changes caused by the fight-or-flight response include increases in blood pressure, heart rate, body metabolism, rate of breathing, and blood flow to the muscles of the arms and legs. The sympathetic nervous system controls this response. Its effects are what we feel each time under stress.

2. Stress results from positive and negative demands.

Many of us have become conditioned to think that stress results only from unpleasant demands. This is false. Research demonstrates that pleasant as well as unpleasant activities cause stress.[2] For example, a kiss or a tennis match will cause a stress reaction in most of us. As such, stress is not necessarily something bad that should be avoided. For many people this is a strange concept.

3. Stress results from mental, as well as physical, demands.

When we think of the fight-or-flight response, we often consider only physical demands like racing to an accident or fleeing from a mugger. But mental demands can cause the same response. Think of the last time you worried about a problem employee or a budget snag. As managers, we face frequent mental demands. Often the stress from mental demands is more difficult to dissipate than the stress from physical demands.

Stress and performance

Think about the last time you "blew up" about something around the house. Perhaps you'd had a difficult day. As you walked through the front door, your husband, wife, or roommate made a relatively minor request of you: "Hey, did you pick up the package I asked you to?" Ordinarily you would have said either yes or no, and the matter would have been closed. But because you had a bad day, because people had been placing many demands on you, you probably said something like "Who do I look like—Federal Express?" You'd had it "up to here." This example highlights a fundamental point: *Your ability to cope with stress depends on the amount of stress to which you are exposed.* This fact is particularly significant when you consider the effects of stress on performance. In 1908 Robert M. Yerkes and John D. Dodson of the Harvard Physiologic Laboratory demonstrated that as stress increases, so does performance, but only up to a critical point.[3] Beyond that point, further stress causes a decrease in performance. This relationship is known as the Yerkes-Dodson curve and is shown in Figure 11–1.

As you can see from the curve, stress can be a positive force leading to increased performance. We all need some stress to perform optimally; without it we become bored and unproductive. Too much stress, however, leads to reduced performance and the downward spiral of burnout. Let's look at how EMS managers describe how it feels to be at particular points on the Yerkes-Dodson curve.

Point A on the Yerkes-Dodson curve is the upslope position. For a person at point A, additional stress would improve performance. When asked to place herself on the Yerkes-Dodson curve, an EMS secretarial supervisor put herself at point A and said: "I'm bored. I'm the type of person who likes to keep busy... I need to have new and different things to handle... to run on high stress, I guess... or I get bored. We've recently been working on some new programming, which was interesting, but then that stopped. The day-to-day work, that's all right, but after a while it gets tedious. You need something to think about... something to tackle and accomplish which isn't your day-to-day stuff. The best thing that could happen to me now would be for someone to walk

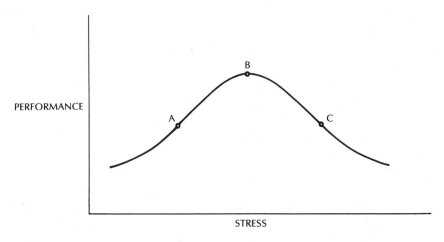

FIGURE 11-1. **Yerkes-Dodson Curve**

in tomorrow morning and throw down a new challenge on my desk."

Point B on the Yerkes-Dodson curve is the peak position. A person at point B would be operating at top efficiency but would have little capacity to cope positively with increased stress. When asked to place herself on the Yerkes-Dodson curve, a nursing supervisor chose point B and said: "I feel like I'm pushing right toward the top. Everything seems to be going in my direction. I rarely feel tired and my mind is going so fast I would like to do about six things at once. I think that in my work situation I need to be careful that I don't push others too hard. They're not at the point I am. They can't be pushed as hard as I'm pushing."

Point C is the downslope, or burnout position, on the Yerkes-Dodson curve. A person at point C would be operating at low efficiency, and increased stress would only make matters worse. When asked to place herself on the Yerkes-Dodson curve, an EMT-ambulance supervisor said: "The way it started is that the petty little things began to bother me, things that in the past I would have let go by. Everything became real important. I began to live and breathe my work. I began to feel that my needs weren't very important. I felt like I was going to lose control. . . . See, you begin to fear that the next guy that comes in the door or calls on the phone is the one who's going to break your back. So you become paranoid—worried that everyone is making demands on you and that you're not going to be able to meet them. Then I had a big personnel problem. I had to terminate a guy who wasn't working out. . . . It was very difficult and the process lasted a long time.   When I finished I was at the end of my rope. The questions start: 'Who am I?' 'Why am I doing what I'm doing?' 'Is it really worth all the trouble?' 'Where do I go from here?' I cried. You know . . . sometimes you're scared you're going crazy. Because you've seen people go through this before and actually break down. Living gets to be a real effort. You feel cheated that you've put all this effort into your work and no one cares. Your productivity is nil. If you do go to work, it becomes a real chore. I've seen people in my position quit . . . often not immediately . . . they just fade out of the picture. I feel real vulnerable. I'll make it back, though, because I have support. You need it. Someone reaching out their hand to you . . . a support system of some sort. If you survive it, you say: 'I never want to have that feeling again.' But unless I change something, I'm going to go back and do it all over."

Determining your level of stress

As you can see from the Yerkes-Dodson curve, once stress reaches a certain point, further increases in stress reduce performance. You need to know when you begin on the down-slope, when you have passed your peak performance so that any additional stress will reduce performance rather than enhance it. This downslope is popularly called *burnout* and is a common problem in EMS management.

Where would you place yourself on the curve? In order to help you identify how much stress you are under, we provide you with the following two exercises.

As mentioned, both good and bad events cause stress. What affects your performance is the total amount of stress that you are experiencing. Think about your life over the last 18 months. How many of the events shown in Table 11–1 have occurred?

Total the score for the stressful events in your life. The higher your score, the farther along you are on the Yerkes-Dodson curve. If your score is above 12, you may be past the point of peak performance on the curve.[4]

TABLE 11–1. Stressful Events

EVENT	Value
1. Death of spouse	5
2. Divorce	4
3. Marital separation	3
4. Death of close family member	3
5. Personal injury or illness	3
6. Marriage	3
7. Fired at work	2
8. Marital reconciliation	2
9. Change in health of family member	2
10. Pregnancy	2
11. Gain of new family member	2
12. Change in financial state	2
13. Death of close friend	2
14. Change to a different line of work	2
15. Change in responsibilities at work	2
16. Son or daughter leaving home	1
17. Outstanding personal achievement	1
18. Begin or end school	1
19. Change in work hours or conditions	1
20. Change in residence	1

One of the weaknesses of the previous list is that it does not list many of the stressful annoyances that face an EMS manager daily. In order to capture these subjective factors, let's look at how your level of stress has affected you emotionally. Ask yourself the following questions:[5]

1. Do you tire easily?
2. Are people telling you, "You don't look so good lately"?
3. Are you working harder and accomplishing less?
4. Are you increasingly cynical and disenchanted?
5. Do you often feel sad without explanation?
6. Are you forgetting things (appointments, deadlines, etc.)?
7. Are you irritable and short-tempered?
8. Are you seeing close friends less frequently?
9. Are you too busy to do even routine things like make phone calls, read reports, or send out Christmas cards?
10. Are you unable to joke or laugh at yourself?
11. Does sex seem as if it's more trouble than it's worth?
12. Do you have little to say to people?

If you answered yes to any of these questions, you may be suffering the negative effects of stress. The more yes answers, the more likely that you are on the downslope of the Yerkes-Dodson curve—burning out.

These two measures don't provide you with a foolproof method of assessing the amount of stress that you are undergoing. Dealing with death on a daily basis, for example, causes a significant amount of stress. So does handling chronic personnel problems. Think about all the events in your professional and personal life that are causing stress. Combine those thoughts with the results of the two exercises that we have given you. Then place yourself on the Yerkes-Dodson curve. Are you like many EMS managers—riding the downslope of burnout? The best place to be on the scale is not at the peak. Being at the peak gives you no resilience to handle unforeseen stresses or emergencies. Your goal should be to be on the upslope of the curve. Leave yourself with a cushion so you can respond to unforeseen stress with increased performance.

Stress and your personality

You probably know people who seem to be able to handle tremendous amounts of stress without any apparent problems. People like that exist, but most of us aren't that lucky. We must look at ways we can make ourselves more resilient to stress. As a first step we must evaluate our personalities, because the quantity of stress that we face is not the sole determinant of whether we will have stress-related problems. Personality type is also important. Friedman and Rosenman first noted the connection between certain personality traits and coronary heart disease in 1959.[6,7] They described two major personality types (type A and type B) who have markedly different responses to stress. Table 11–2 describes the characteristics of each personality type.

It is important that you know whether you are a type A personality: ambitious, competitive, impatient, and unable to relax. One way to find out is to ask yourself the following questions:[8]

1. Do you walk, eat, and move rapidly?
2. Do you become angry when you are in slow lines or in traffic?
3. Do you generally feel impatient?
4. Do you do two or more things simultaneously?
5. Do you feel guilty if you relax or take a vacation?
6. Do you think about other things when you are talking to someone?

TABLE 11–2. Type A and Type B Personality Traits

THE TYPE A PERSONALITY	THE TYPE B PERSONALITY
Displays excessive competitive drive.	Is able to play for fun.
Is ambitious and achievement-oriented	Has no need to display achievements.
Tries to do many things at once.	Works for quality not quantity.
Is greatly concerned with meeting deadlines; is impatient.	Displays no sense of urgency.
Is unable to relax without feeling guilty.	Can relax without feeling guilty.

7. Do you work hurriedly, even if there is no deadline?

8. Do you continue to assume more responsibility, even when you are having difficulty managing current responsibilities?

9. Do you have nervous gestures, like grinding your teeth, clenching your fists, or drumming your fingers?

10. Do you commit yourself to activities when you know you don't have the time for them?

These are some of the characteristics of type A people. If you answered yes to more than seven of these questions, you may have a type A personality.

The health consequences of type A behavior are serious. In coronary heart disease the magnitude of type A risk is roughly equal to that of high blood pressure or smoking.[9] This fact makes clear the need to control type A behavior if you are going to pursue a high-stress job like EMS management and survive.

Controlling stress

By now you should know where you sit on the Yerkes-Dodson curve and what your personality type is. If you are a type A personality or on the downslope of the curve, learning to control stress is a critical issue. Even if you are type B or on the upslope of the curve, learning to control stress is still important, because you are likely to have periods when your stress demands escalate and you must be prepared to handle them.

Let's examine four general approaches to dealing with stress: combatting overwork, meditation, exercise, and controlling worry.

Combatting overwork

Unfortunately for many EMS managers periods of overwork are a fact of life. You'll be able to eliminate most of your overwork by using the effective time management techniques outlined in Chapter 1. Despite your efforts, however, you are likely to face occasional periods of 60-hour workweeks. Those managers at greatest risk for overwork are those who combine clinical work with management. For example, an EMT-manager may carefully plan 40-hour administrative workweeks. The loss of a staff EMT may force that EMT-manager to provide 40 hours a week of

direct patient care until a replacement EMT can be found. During
that period the EMT-manager must continue his administrative
work. As a result his carefully planned 40-hour workweeks will
expand to 60, 70, or 80 hours. Many EMS managers face this risk
of overwork.

Some managers can effectively cope with overwork. Others
can't. Can we learn anything by studying the characteristics of
those professionals who can effectively cope with periods of
overwork?[10] Table 11–3 summarizes the differences between
those professionals who can and those who can't.

Professionals who effectively cope with overwork respond
to fatigue by taking time off. They have the ability to suppress
thinking about problems until an appropriate time to deal with
them. In addition, they exercise regularly, enjoy vacations, have a
stable family situation, maintain friendships, and avoid chemical
dependence. One thing that you'll notice when you read the list is
that some of the characteristics of those people who can't cope
with overwork are similar to the characteristics of people on the
downslope of the Yerkes-Dodson curve, for example, lengthening
the day to compensate for diminished productivity and an inabil-
ity to laugh at oneself. This illustrates an important point: If you
expect to thrive on long work hours, you must build and maintain

TABLE 11–3. Differences Between Those Professionals Who Effectively Cope With Overwork and Those Who Don't

THE PROFESSIONAL WHO COPES	THE PROFESSIONAL WHO CAN'T COPE
Can postpone thinking about problems.	Ruminates about work problems.
Is able to respond promptly to fatigue.	Lengthens workday to compensate for diminished productivity.
Avoids chemical abuse.	Uses alcohol and drugs as an escape from stress.
Schedules vacations.	Tends to postpone vacations.
Has stable domestic situation.	Has chaotic family life.
Is able to maintain friendships.	Is a loner.
Engages in regular exercise.	Has sedentary life style.
Has varied interests outside work.	Has narrowed interests.
Displays sense of humor.	Is unable to laugh at self.

a reserve capacity to handle unexpected stress. You cannot try to operate at full throttle, peak efficiency all of the time.

Let's take a moment to discuss drug and alcohol abuse. Don't kid yourself into believing that drug and alcohol dependency is something that happens to *other* people. Health care providers have higher than average rates of chemical abuse. EMS managers provide health care for long hours under high stress. Under these circumstances alcohol and drug abuse can easily occur. Is it a problem for you? One way to find out is to ask yourself these questions:[11]

- Have you ever felt that you should cut down on your drinking or drug use?
- Have people annoyed you by criticizing your drinking or drug use?
- Have you ever had a drink first thing in the morning to steady your nerves or get rid of a hangover?
- Have you ever felt bad or guilty about your drinking or drug use?

If you answered yes to two questions, you are likely to have a problem with chemical abuse. If you answered yes to three or four questions, you almost certainly have a problem with chemical abuse.

Meditation

Meditation sounds like a fad, but if you dismiss meditation as a means of controlling stress, you'll miss one of the most effective, time- and science-proven stress reducers.

Although meditation can make you more relaxed in general, it is particularly valuable in countering the dangerous effects of stress on the cardiovascular system. As described earlier, stress (or the fight-or-flight response) occurs when the brain perceives a threat in the environment and activates the sympathetic nervous system, which in turn increases heart rate and blood pressure. This can have serious consequences, particularly if your sympathetic nervous system is stimulated frequently during the day in response to physical or emotional stressors. Blood pressure that is frequently elevated during the day during stress responses tends to remain at permanently elevated levels. This can lead to an increased risk of heart attack and stroke. Heart attack is the primary mechanism by which stress kills.

Meditation counters this sequence, inhibiting the sympathetic nervous system so that heart rate and blood pressure decrease. Meditation can cause permanent reductions in blood pressure. Thus meditation both reduces the immediate psychic effects of stress by promoting relaxation and counteracts the long-term physical effects by reducing the risk of stroke and heart attack.

There are numerous kinds of meditation and meditationlike activities: transcendental meditation, Zen, Yoga, autogenic training, progressive relaxation, and hypnosis with suggested deep relaxation. Herbert Bensen, M.D., combined key features from time-proven meditation practices into a technique called the *relaxation response*.[12] He used the relaxation response with people suffering from high blood pressure and found that those people were able to lower their systolic blood pressure an average of 10 millimeters of mercury. Although the relaxation response is relatively simple to evoke, you must learn several key steps to use it effectively. (Because the response represents an altered state of consciousness, it is difficult to produce spontaneously.) Dr. Bensen notes four basic elements of the relaxation response.

1. **Quiet environment.** You should select as calm or quiet an environment as possible. An unused room or an isolated outdoor setting works well.

2. **Mental device.** You must free your mind from the purposeful, problem-solving track that it normally follows. Most of us are unable to think of nothing; our minds wander. A mental device—repeating a word or phrase, concentrating on a focal point, or concentrating on your breathing—will help you break away from your purposeful thoughts without having your mind wander.

3. **Passive attitude.** Despite your efforts to free your mind, distracting thoughts will occur. Don't criticize yourself for having distracting thoughts. Instead, as soon as you become aware that your mind has wandered, redirect yourself to your mental device. Don't worry about performing your technique perfectly.

4. **Comfortable position.** Generally, lying down is not a good idea because you are likely to fall asleep. A comfortable sitting position, however, is essential if you are to avoid muscle tension; reclining chairs work well.

The specifics of technique will vary from person to person. One effective method follows:

1. Wait at least two hours after eating because the digestive process seems to interfere with the response.
2. Sit down in a reclining chair in a quiet, unoccupied, darkened room.
3. Remove your shoes and any constricting clothing (tie, vest, sweater, etc.).
4. Close your eyes.
5. Beginning at your feet, tense and relax all your muscles—one group at a time, from your toes to your forehead.
6. Concentrate on your breathing. Breathe deeply through your nose. While you are breathing, count to yourself ("In...1...2...3...4...out...1...2...3...4..."). If it helps, visualize a peaceful setting while breathing—a secluded beach or a calm pool of water are helpful images.
7. Continue this for about 20 minutes.
8. Open your eyes. Sit quietly for a few minutes.

Let's be honest. When first presented with the concept of meditation, you may think it a little far-fetched. But if you're willing to keep an open mind about experimenting with meditation, you'll probably be pleasantly surprised with how fast you can master it.

Exercise

Exercise has a double impact on stress. First, exercise makes you more relaxed and better able to cope with stress. Second, exercise improves your cardiovascular fitness so that you become less likely to suffer cardiovascular disease.

Why does exercise make us feel better? Although the reasons are poorly understood, evidence is emerging to indicate that exercise causes fundamental changes in our body chemistry that relate to mood.[13,14] Endorphins, morphinelike substances that occur in the body, affect our mood, resistance to pain, appetite, thermoregulation, and sleep. Exercise training causes an increase in endorphins in our bloodstream. While we must learn much more about these substances, it is clear that exercise causes a change in endorphin levels, which leads to basic physiological and psychological changes producing greater pain tolerance and relaxation.

While the exact nature of the effect of exercise on mood is uncertain, the effect of exercise on cardiovascular fitness is certain: Exercise reduces your risk of heart attack. If you manage in EMS, you should know what your cardiovascular disease risk is and develop an exercise program, not only to reduce your cardiac risk but to help combat stress as well.

There are many models to determine cardiac risk. Here is a simple one:[15]

1. If either of your parents died of heart disease, high blood pressure, or stroke before the age of 60, give yourself 6 points.

2. If you smoke a pack of cigarettes or more a day, give yourself 10 points. If you smoke less than a pack a day, give yourself 4 points. If you don't smoke, you get 0.

3. Count your pulse for 15 seconds. If 23 or greater, you get 5 points. If 20 to 22, you get 2 points. If less than 20, you get 0.

4. Calculate your ideal weight. (For men: 106 pounds plus 6 pounds for every inch over 5 feet. For women: 100 pounds plus 5 pounds for every inch over 5 feet. For example, a 6-foot man would have an ideal weight of 178.) Calculate the percentage that you are over or under your ideal weight. To do this, subtract your ideal weight from your current weight, multiply by 100, then divide by your ideal weight. For example, a 200-pound, 6-foot man would be $(200 - 178) \times 100/178$ or 12 percent overweight. If you are more than 25 percent overweight, give yourself 3 points; between 5 percent underweight and 25 percent overweight, 2 points; more than 5 percent underweight, 0.

5. Determine your diastolic blood pressure. If it is 110 or greater, you get 8 points. If it is 95 to 109, you get 2 points. If 90 to 94, you get 1 point. If less than 90, you get 0.

6. Now total your score.
   0–2   Group 1—lowest risk group
   3–6   Group 2—risk 1.5 times higher than group 1

7–10   Group 3—risk 2.5 times higher than group 1
11–13   Group 4—risk 3 times higher than group 1
14–30   Group 5—risk 4.5 times higher than group 1

If you smoke a pack of cigarettes a day, are more than 25 percent overweight, and have a 15-second pulse of 23, your risk of coronary disease is more than 4.5 times higher than if you stopped smoking and exercised to reduce your weight and pulse. An exercise program is important for all EMS managers. It is particularly important, however, for those managers in the high coronary-risk groups.

When we talk about exercise programs to increase your tolerance for stress, we are referring to aerobic exercise programs. Aerobic exercise enables a greater amount of oxygen to reach your body tissues. Remember how stress operates. Through repeated stimulation of the sympathetic nervous system, stress causes hypertension, which can lead to decreased blood flow to the heart and brain. Through an aerobic exercise program, you can counteract this deadly process. Specifically aerobic exercise does the following:

1.   Enables the lungs to process more air.
2.   Increases the oxygen-carrying capacity of the blood.
3.   Increases blood flow at lower blood pressures.
4.   Strengthens the heart and increases its reserve for periods of high output.

These changes increase your ability to deliver oxygen to your vital organs. This extra capacity is important when your fight-or-flight response is being repeatedly stimulated. Under these conditions the stronger your heart and the greater your capacity to deliver oxygen to your body, the safer you are. Examples of aerobic exercises include dancing, walking, running, lap swimming, and bicycling. The two chief characteristics of these aerobic exercises are that they are *vigorous* and *sustained*. Nonaerobic exercises do not appreciably benefit the heart and the lungs. Examples are sprinting, golf, bowling, baseball, doubles tennis, and isometrics.

Remember: Exercise is important as both a stress reducer and a cardiovascular conditioner. If you are a type A personality, a high cardiac risk, or in poor physical condition, begin planning your exercise program now. First check with your physician to find out at what level you can safely begin such a program. Then

pull out your schedule for the next month. When could you exercise? What will you do? Also plan to read a good book on
exercise.[16]

Controlling worry

What do you have to worry about? If you are an EMS manager,
your budget is probably in trouble, your work schedule looks
shaky, one of your ambulances may break down at any time, your
presentation for a conference next week is not complete, and on
and on. Worry—it can be a major cause of stress for many
managers. How do you overcome it? There is no single answer.
Although different strategies work in different situations, try to
adopt these five rules into your daily living.[17]

Rule 1. Live in day-tight compartments.

Concentrate on the work that you have at hand. Often worry
results from excessive concern with the future. Planning for the
future *is* important, but you meet your goals one day at a time.
Make out your daily to-do list and follow it. You'll find the long-
term goals will be accomplished without your worrying about
them.

Rule 2. When presented with serious trouble, ask, "What is the worst that can happen?"

It's Christmas Eve and one of your staff calls in sick. Immediately you worry, "What am I going to do?" Whenever potentially
serious trouble comes up, ask yourself, "What is the worst that
can happen?" Are you going to die? No. Are you going to lose your
job? No. Might you end up having to work Christmas Eve?
Perhaps. Accept the worst and prepare yourself mentally to deal
with it.

Rule 3. Before you start worrying about something, be sure of the facts.

You arrive at work one morning and are told that your staff
picked up the mayor's son following a bicycle accident and swore

at the mayor. Is this a real problem? Sure it is, if the mayor signs your checks and *if it really happened.* A great deal of worry can be caused by events that never occurred or by statements taken out of context. Whenever you are presented with a particularly stressful accusation, dig out the facts *first.* Once you have them, ask yourself the following:

- What is the problem?
- What is the cause of the problem?
- What are all possible solutions?
- What is the best possible solution?

Once you know what the best possible solution is, carry it out.

Rule 4. Accept the inevitable.

If the state enacts a regulation that every EMT must take a refresher course every 18 months, and you think that such a regulation is unreasonable, fight it. However, if you fight the regulation and lose, accept the inevitable. There is nothing to be gained from worrying about events that you cannot control.

Rule 5. Don't try to relive the past.

If you are a manager, recognize that you are human and that you will make mistakes from time to time. When something goes wrong, it's human nature to second-guess yourself. Perhaps you terminate a problem employee and later wonder whether the facts on which you based your decision were erroneous, or you manage a difficult medical case that has a bad outcome and you try to figure out a way that you could have handled things differently. When things don't go as well as you think they should, analyze what you have done so that you will do better next time. Then move on. Don't try to relive the past; you can't.

If you can control worry, cope with periods of overwork, practice relaxation techniques, and exercise vigorously, you can limit the effect that stress will have upon you. As a manager, however, you must also control the impact that stress is having on your coworkers. Try to educate them in the techniques that we have outlined here.

Stress and the organization

Organizations and managers contribute to the stress of employees. As a manager, you must not contribute to the problem by being a stress carrier. Do the following stress-causing characteristics exist in your service?

RESPONSIBILITY WITHOUT AUTHORITY AND CONTROL. When you delegate tasks to your subordinates, make sure that you give them enough authority to complete the task successfully. Delegation works best when the delegated authority is adequate to meet the delegated responsibility. However, if the authority is lacking or when control of the outcome is impossible, stress can result. For example, if you want a subordinate to develop the most effective way of packing a jump kit, don't saddle that person with assorted rules about what must and must not be packed. Some organizations are stress-ridden because the top manager clings to all authority. Encourage yourself and those around you to delegate adequate authority.

TIME PRESSURE. Some time pressure cannot be changed. You must start CPR within seven minutes to prevent brain death, for example. But many times deadlines are arbitrary. Don't impose unrealistic deadlines on yourself or others.

LACK OF JOB CLARITY. A simple task, like answering the telephone in an emergency department, can cause stress if the secretaries think that the nurses are supposed to do it and the nurses think the secretaries are supposed to do it. Make sure that job responsibilities are clear for your subordinates. If you find yourself bumping heads with a coworker in some area, discuss the task and reach a compromise.

CONFRONTING NUMEROUS PROBLEMS. When you first assume a management job, numerous problems confront you. Unless you establish priorities among those problems, you will be subject to the ongoing stress of not knowing which pressing matter to handle next.

CHAOTIC PROCEDURES. Change is stressful. Healthy people often resist change, so don't constantly change rules and procedures; that just leads to chaos and increased stress.

POOR COMMUNICATION. Poor communication keeps employees in the dark about what is expected of them and denies them feedback regarding how they are doing. This uncertainty causes stress. As much as possible, keep people informed about all events that relate to their positions.

Summary

This chapter can assist you in learning more about yourself and the effects of stress on you. By now you should know what stress is and how it affects performance, where you sit on the Yerkes-Dodson curve, and whether you are running the risk of burning out. You should understand your personality type and its consequences for the impact of stress on your health. You should know what your physical condition is, how you can combat stress and worry, and how you can avoid being a stress-carrying manager. This chapter contains several exercises because you must take an active role if you are to be effective in managing your stress. Unless you learn to manage stress, all other management skills are meaningless, because you won't be in EMS management long enough to use them.

Epilogue

If you have reached this point without detour, you are now familiar with a core of material that is critical for effective management in emergency medical services. This book hasn't provided you with the details of different ambulance types or places where you can buy the best radios. Facts like that change. Your ability to remember such facts won't determine whether you succeed or fail as a manager. Rather, the effective EMS manager is distinguished from the ineffective one by the ability to think. This book teaches you to think like a manager.

If we can leave you with one summarizing principle, it's this: Successful managers think before they act. For EMS managers this is often difficult. After all, we've been geared to handling emergencies, where the key element has been to act *fast*. In a crisis the right decision, if not implemented quickly enough, becomes the wrong decision. In EMS management, on the other hand, there is little incentive for making split-second decisions. The important thing is to make the decision correctly. As an EMS manager, you must recognize that taking the time to think a problem through and examine all possible solutions is not a luxury, it's a necessity.

This book demonstrates how to plan, organize, direct, control, and survive in EMS management. Don't expect to develop these skills overnight; they require practice. They are rarely applied the same way in any two situations. Ask effective EMS managers exactly what they do, and they will probably say that every day is different from the previous ones. Should this disillusion you, probe further. They'll probably add that the ever-changing EMS environment is the key to the challenge and satisfaction of the work.

It would be nice if simply reading a book could assure your success as a manager, but unfortunately it's not that easy. In addition to understanding the principles and techniques that we have presented, you must gain practice in applying them. Managing your time wisely, listening to others effectively, appraising the members of your service—these skills all require repeated use in order to be sharpened. Our goal has been to point you in the right direction so you can avoid some of the mistakes of ourselves and others. It's up to you to put these principles into practice.

Notes

Chapter 1

1. Portions of this chapter previously appeared in "Time Management: A Survival Guide for EMS Managers" by W. L. Newkirk, *Emergency Medical Services* 10, no. 5 (1981): 68–72.
2. Clarence Randall, *The Folklore of Management* (Boston: Little, Brown, 1961), 120–28.
3. Alan Lakein, *How to Get Control of Your Time and Your Life* (New York: New American Library, 1974), 30–36.
4. R. Alec Mackenzie, *The Time Trap* (New York: McGraw-Hill, 1972), 51–53.
5. Ibid., 38–39.
6. The idea of a timewasters analysis is not original with this chapter; see R. Alec Mackenzie, *Managing at the Top* (New York: The President's Association, 1970).

Chapter 2

1. John B. Lasagna, "Make Your MBO Pragmatic," *Harvard Business Review* 49, no. 6 (1971): 64–69.
2. Peter F. Drucker, *Management: Tasks, Responsibilities, Practices* (New York: Harper and Row, 1974).
3. Ibid., 431.
4. John Wally, M.D., and William Barnum adapted the priority planning system from United Parcel Service to running their emergency medical corporation in the early 1970s. This was one of the earliest adaptations of priority planning to emergency medicine.
5. William L. Newkirk, M.D., "Managing for Motivation in EMS," *Emergency Medical Services* 9, no. 3 (1980): 50–56.
6. Abraham H. Maslow, *Motivation and Personality* (New York: Harper and Row, 1970).
7. F. Herzberg, "One More Time: How Do You Motivate Employees?" In *Harvard Business Review: On Management* (New York: Harper and Row, 1975).
8. Ian G. Rawson et al., "A Formal Approach to Planning for a County Level EMS System," *Emergency Medical Services* 10, no. 2 (1981): 60–69.

Chapter 3

1. Ernest Dale, *Management: Theory and Practice* (New York: McGraw-Hill, 1969).

2. Alan C. Filley and Robert J. House, *Managerial Process and Organizational Behavior* (Glenview, IL: Scott, Foresman and Company, 1964).

3. Charles T. Horngren, *Cost Accounting: A Managerial Emphasis* (Englewood Cliffs: Prentice-Hall, 1972), 244–50.

4. K. Patricia Cross, *Adults as Learners* (San Francisco: Jossey Bass, 1981).

5. Linda K. Bock, *Teaching Adults in Continuing Education* (Urbana: University of Illinois, 1979).

6. These observations on EMS education stem from discussions with Patrick Cote, RN, EMT, director of EMS education/training of the state of Maine. Mr. Cote has directed the training of over 5,000 EMS personnel. He is also on the U.S. Department of Transportation's Paramedic Committee.

7. Madge Atwood, "Teacher Training for EMT-A Instructors in Illinois," *Emergency Medical Services* 11, no. 3 (1982): 71–81.

Chapter 4

1. A portion of this chapter appeared previously as W. L. Newkirk, "Managing the Aftermath of Rapid EMS Growth: What Happens When the Federal Funds Dry Up?" *Emergency Medical Services* 9, no. 6 (1980): 123–26.

2. Maryland Hospital Education Institute, *Hospital Sponsored Ambulatory Care* (Chicago: American Hospital Association, 1980), 48–49.

3. Ibid., 39–43.

4. Harry V. Roberts, *Conversational Statistics* (Palo Alto, CA: Scientific Press, 1974).

Chapter 5

1. A portion of this chapter appeared in W. L. Newkirk and Richard Linden, "EMS Management: Improving Communication through Active Listening," *Emergency Medical Services* 11, no. 7 (1982): 8–11.

2. Leon Festinger, "Cognitive Dissonance," *Scientific American* 207, no. 4 (1962): 93–102.

3. Carl Rogers and Richard Farson, "Active Listening" in *Communication and Organizational Behavior,* edited by William Harey (Homewood, IL: R. D. Irwin, 1967), 81–97.

4. Carl Rogers and F. J. Roethlisberger, "Barriers and Gateways to Communication," *Harvard Business Review,* 30, no. 4 (1952): 46–52.

5. Robert Burns, *The Listening Techniques* (Chicago: University of Chicago, 1958).

6. William Morris, Ed., *American Heritage Dictionary of the English Language,* s.v. "Assert." (New York: Houghton-Mifflin, 1970), p. 79.

7. Sharon A. Bower and Gordon H. Bower, *Asserting Yourself* (Reading, MA: Addison Wesley, 1976).

8. Manuel T. Smith, *When I Say "No," I Feel Guilty* (New York: Bantam Books, 1975).

Chapter 6

1. Some of this chapter previously appeared as W. L. Newkirk, "Cooperative Negotiations: The Key to Getting What You Need in EMS," *Emergency Medical Services* 10, no. 3 (1981): 30–36.

2. J. Z. Rubin and B. R. Brown, *The Social Psychology of Bargaining and Negotiation* (New York: Academic Press, 1975).

3. A. H. Maslow, *Motivation and Personality* (New York: Harper and Row, 1970), 35–39.

4. Peter B. Laubach et al., *Process, Art, and Technique of Negotiating* (Chicago: American College of Hospital Administrators, 1977), 25–26.

5. T. Shelling, "An Essay on Bargaining" in *Bargaining: Formal Theories of Negotiation,* edited by O. Young (Urbana: University of Illinois, 1975), 319–42.

Chapter 7

1. William Newman and Charles Summer, *The Process of Management* (Englewood Cliffs: Prentice-Hall, 1961), 58–75.

2. Mackenzie, op. cit., 123–24.

3. Newman and Summer, op. cit., 58–75.

4. Mackenzie, op. cit., 136.

5. Alvin Brown, *Organization of Industry* (Englewood Cliffs NJ: Prentice-Hall, 1947), 27–46.

6. William Oncken and Donald Wass, "Management Time: Who's Got the Monkey?" *Harvard Business Review,* November–December 1974, 10–17.

Chapter 8

1. A portion of this chapter appeared previously as W. L. Newkirk, "Managing the Aftermath of Rapid EMS Growth: What Happens When the Federal Funds Dry Up?" *Emergency Medical Services* 9, no. 6 (1980): 123–26.

2. Sheldon Glass, *Life-Control: How to Assert Leadership in Any Situation* (New York: Evans, 1976).

3. J. P. Kotter and L. A. Schlesinger, "Choosing Strategies for Change," *Harvard Business Review* 57 (1979): 106–14.

4. J. P. Kotter, *Power in Management* (New York: Anacom, 1979).

5. D. C. McClelland and D. H. Burnham, "Power Is the Great Motivator," *Harvard Business Review* 54 (1976): 100–10.

Chapter 9

1. Ellen M. Lerch, "Criteria-Based Performance Appraisals," *Nursing Management* 13, no. 7 (1982): 28–31.

2. Robert F. Mager and Peter Pipe, *Analyzing Performance Problems* (Belmont, CA: Pitman Learning, 1970).

3. Lester R. Bittel, *What Every Supervisor Should Know* (Englewood Cliffs NJ: Prentice-Hall, 1968), 133–43.

4. William Davidson, *How to Develop and Administer an Effective Wage and Salary Program* (Chicago: Dartnell, 1974), 199–232.

5. William Marshall, *Administering the Company Personnel Function* (Englewood Cliffs: Prentice-Hall, 1976), 79–88.

6. Dallas-Fort Worth Hospital Council, *Coping with the Joint Commission: Quality Assurance* (Dallas: Dallas-Fort Worth Hospital Council, 1982).

Chapter 10

1. Charles Horngren, *Cost Accounting: A Managerial Emphasis* (Englewood Cliffs: Prentice-Hall, 1972), 160.

Chapter 11

1. Dr. Cannon discusses his findings on the sympathetic nervous system in Walter B. Cannon and Arturo Rosenblueth, *Autonomic Neuroeffector Systems* (New York: Macmillan, 1937).

2. H. Selye, *The Stress of Life* (New York: McGraw-Hill, 1976).

3. H. Bensen and R. Allen, "How Much Stress Is Too Much?" *Harvard Business Review*, September–October 1980, 86–92.

4. This stress events rating scale is based on a widely used scale called the Holmes Life Events Scale.

5. These questions are derived from a series of burnout-related questions in H. Freudenberger, *Burn-out* (Garden City: Anchor Press, 1980).

6. M. Friedman and R. H. Rosenman, "Association of Specific Overt Behavior Pattern with Blood and Cardiovascular Findings: Blood Cholesterol Level, Blood Clotting Time, Incidence of Arcus Senilis and Clinical Coronary Artery Disease," *Journal of the American Medical Association* 169 (1959): 1286–96.

7. R. Rosenman et al., "Coronary Heart Disease in the Western Collaborative Group Study. Final Follow-up Experience of 8½ Years," *Journal of the American Medical Association* 233 (1975): 872–77.

8. These type A personality questions are derived from a list by P. W. Buffington, "An Anti-Stress Survival Kit," *Sky*, April 1983, 85–87.

9. "Coronary Prone Behavior and Coronary Heart Disease: A Critical Review." *Circulation* 63 (1981): 1199–215.

10. J. I. Walker, "Prescription for the Stressed Physician," *Behavioral Medicine*, September 1980, 12–17.

11. D. Mayfield et al., "The CAGE Questionnaire: Validation of a New Alcoholism Screening Instrument," *American Journal of Psychiatry* 131, no. 10 (1974): 1121–23.

12. H. Bensen, *The Relaxation Response* (New York: Avon, 1975).

13. D. B. Carr et al., "Physical Conditioning Facilitates the Exercise-Induced Secretion of Beta-Endorphin and Beta-Lipotropin in Women," *New England Journal of Medicine* 305 (1981): 560–63.

14. O. Appenzeller, "What Makes Us Run?" *New England Journal of Medicine* 305 (1981): 578–80.

15. Alan R. Dyer et al. "A Self-Scoring Five-Question Risk Test for Coronary Heart Disease," *Circulation* 60 (1979): 914.

16. K. Cooper, *Aerobics* (New York: Bantam, 1968).

17. D. Carnegie, *How to Stop Worrying and Start Living* (New York: Pocket Books, 1953).

Other sources

American Association of Industrial Management. *Job Rating Manual.* Dedham, MA: American Association of Industrial Management, 1969.

Atkinson, J. W., and L. Raynor. *Motivation and Achievement.* Washington: Winston and Sons, 1974.

Behrman, Edward A. *Hospital Purchasing.* St. Louis: Catholic Hospital Association, 1982.

Benton, A. A., et al. "Effects of Extremity of Offers and Concession Rate on Outcomes of Bargaining," *Journal of Personality and Social Psychiatry,* 24 (1972): 73–83.

Berman, Howard J., and Lewis E. Weeks. *The Financial Management of Hospitals.* Ann Arbor: Health Administration Press, 1982.

Binis, Raymond. "The Performance Appraisal: The Most Needed and Neglected Management Tool," *Supervisory Management,* October 1978, 12–16.

California Hospital Association. *Budgeting Manual.* Sacramento: California Hospital Association, 1977.

Cross, K. Patricia. *Accent on Learning.* San Francisco: Jossey-Bass, 1976.

Deutsch, Karl W. *The Nerves of Government.* London: Free Press of Glencoe, 1963.

Grieff, Barrie S., and Preston K. Munter. *Tradeoffs.* New York: New American Library, 1980.

Hunt, J., and J. Hill. "The New Look in Motivation Theory for Organizational Research," *Human Organization* 28, no. 2 (1969): 100–09.

Jay, Anthony. *Management and Machiavelli.* New York: Holt, Rinehart and Winston, 1967.

Kellogg, Marion S. *Putting Management Theories to Work.* Englewood Cliffs: Prentice-Hall, 1979.

Kelly, Joe. *How Managers Manage.* Englewood Cliffs: Prentice-Hall, 1980.

Kotter, J. P. "Power, Dependence and Effective Management," *Harvard Business Review* 55 (1977): 125–36.

Longenecker, Justin. *Principles of Management and Organizational Behavior.* Columbus: Charles E. Merrill, 1973.

McGregor, D. "The Human Side of Enterprise." In G. W. Dalton and P. R. Lawrence (eds), *Motivation and Control of Organizations.* Homewood, IL: Dorsey Press, 1974, 304–12.

Newman, William. *Administrative Action.* Englewood Cliffs NJ: Prentice-Hall, 1950.

Nierenberg, Gerald I. *The Art of Negotiating.* New York: Cornerstone Library, 1968.

Pascale, Richard T., and Anthony G. Anthos. *The Art of Japanese Management.* New York: Simon and Schuster, 1981.

Porter, L. W., and E. E. Lawler, Jr. "What Job Attitudes Tell About Motivation," *Harvard Business Review,* January–February 1968, 118–26.

Sanders, Norman. *President's Guide to Attracting and Developing Top–Caliber Employees.* Englewood Cliffs: Executive Reports Corporation, 1981.

Schleh, Edward. *Successful Executive Action.* Englewood Cliffs: Prentice-Hall, 1955.

Van Horne, James C. *Financial Management and Policy.* Englewood Cliffs: Prentice-Hall, 1974.

Voluntary Budget Review Organization. *Sample Budgeting Manual.* Augusta ME: Voluntary Budget Review Organization, 1978.

Warshaw, Leon J. *Managing Stress.* Reading: Addison-Wesley, 1979.

Zaleznik, A., et al. *The Motivation, Productivity, and Satisfaction of Workers.* Boston: Harvard University Press, 1958.

Index